THE FITNESS BOOK

Bud Getchell, Ph.D.
Executive Director
The National Institute for Fitness and Sport

Benchmark Press, Inc.
Indianapolis, Indiana

Library of Congress Cataloging in Publication Data:

GETCHELL, BUD 1934-

THE FITNESS BOOK

Cover Design: Gary Schmitt

Art: Craig Gosling

Library of Congress Catalog Card number: 86-71387

ISBN: 0-936157-07-0

Printed in the United States of America
10 9 8 7 6 5 4 3 2 1

The Publisher and Author disclaim responsibility for any adverse effects or consequences from the misapplication or injudicious use of the information contained within this text.

Contents

Part II Moderately Intense Exercise

Part III   Other Fitness Concerns

Acknowledgements

From the start *The Fitness Book* has been a collaboration of efforts by the staff of The National Institute for Fitness and Sport along with assistance from colleagues in the fields of exercise physiology and health promotion. Many people have been involved in searching the current literature and helping to update the information presented in this book.

Assistance from staff members at the Institute include Thomas M. Whitehead, Ed.D., director of The Center for Health and Fitness Programming. Prior to joining the Institute in 1986, Tom was the former Program Director for Fitness at St. Vincent Hospital and Health Care Centers in Indianapolis. He is an ACSM-certified Health/Fitness Instructor and has passed the first phase of ACSM's certification for Health/Fitness Director. Tom recently completed his doctorate of education in adult and community education from Ball State University.

Constance Reardon has brought to the Institute an enthusiasm for fitness and nutrition that is evident daily as she works with participants. She received her M.S. in exercise physiology from Ball State University in 1986 and is an ACSM-certified exercise specialist.

Kay Allen serves as coordinator of special projects at the Institute and heads the internship program. Prior to coming to the Institute in 1986, Kay directed the Adult Fitness Program at the Human Performance Lab at Ball State University. An ACSM-certified Health/Fitness Instructor, Kay has successfully completed the first phase of ACSM's certification for Health/Fitness Director.

Mike Marshall has been involved in corporate health promotion over the past seven years. Prior to joining the Institute, he served as project manager for the Lifewise Programs for Healthy Lifestyles at St. Luke's Hospital in Kansas City, Missouri. Mike was recently awarded an American Lung Association of Indiana fellowship at Indiana University. His expertise in stress management and health promotion has been invaluable during these formulative days at the Institute.

Prior to joining the Institute in 1986, Chris Miller, Ph.D., the Institute's communications' manager, taught journalism and mass communications at Indiana University, Loyola University of the South, and the University of Alabama. She served as the coordinator for the book and was responsible for putting it together in the final form.

The following people have provided specific assistance when needed: David Craig, athletic trainer for the Indiana Pacers; Bob Anderson, author of *Stretching*; and Bill Baun, manager, Health and Fitness, Tenneco, Inc. Two of the Institute's interns also provided expertise: Nanette Dum, R.D., currently working on her Masters in preventive and rehabilitative exercise at Indiana University, reviewed materials for the chapter on Weight Management; and Nancy Moore, whose research on low-impact aerobics was incorporated into Chapter 10, was awarded her Masters in 1987 in exercise physiology from Ball State University. Special thanks for administrative assistance and support goes to Lori Hefner and Nancy Reid.

As an administrator there is never enough time to keep abreast of the current literature. Dialogues with exercise physiologists from around the country were most helpful. Such professionals as David L. Costill, Ph.D.; Jack Wilmore, Ph.D.; Carl Foster, Ph.D.; and Janet P. Wallace, Ph.D. were just a phone call away.

And finally, turning over the working manuscript to our capable editor Kendal Gladish and publisher Butch Cooper was a joy. Kendal's objective editorial skills have polished *The Fitness Book* from a rough gem into a useful, intelligent "how-to" text.

My thanks to each of you.
Bud Getchell

Preface

The foundation of this book is exercise. The key ingredient to total well being is regular exercise. Being physically fit is the positive "do" to good health. This does not mean that exercise is a panacea. It means we need regular exercise as we need food, rest, and sleep to provide groundwork for optimal physiological health and the ability to enjoy a full life.

This book is more than a "how-to" book. It represents the National Institute for Fitness and Sport's philosophy about exercise and its integral role in everyday living. Each page offers you simple basics steps for taking personal responsiblity for overall fitness. It is written for those who want or need help in beginning a fitness program as well as for individuals currently enrolled in an ongoing exercise program at a private club, community center or a corporate-sponsored center.

The simplicity of this book may surprise you. Teaching physical fitness by the page is not easy. Some detailed exercise physiological information has been purposely left out. The most effective instruction calls for personal attention. Throughout the book we encourage you to become involved in a quality program with qualified instructors in your community. If this is not possible, then we are confident the information on these pages is all you need to get started.

This book represents a sifting of the current knowledge that the staff and faculty at the National Institute for Fitness and Sport have acquired from personal involvement in directing and leading exercise and wellness programs over the years. Much of the information is derived from the book *Being Fit* by the Institute's executive director.

There are no gimmicks to physical fitness. Fitness requires your willingness to read and follow the instructions and suggestions set forth. You must be willing to commit yourself to the time and effort it takes to become physically fit. A regular exercise program can be the best investment you ever make. We cannot guarantee you will live longer, but you will be able to do more things with quality in the years to come. Fitness means having the robust health to fully appreciate the joys of life.

Indianapolis, Indiana   Bud Getchell, Ph.D.
June, 1987

Part I

Background

The main ingredient to overall physical fitness is a regular program of cardiorespiratory exercise, a strengthening and conditioning program, and good nutrition. The first three chapters examine physical fitness and how your body responds to exercise. Before undertaking any exercise program, it is important to know just how fit you are. Whether you self-test or undergo a gradual exercise tolerance test, knowing your current level of fitness is important.

Once you have an understanding of your fitness status, it is time to begin a fitness program. Chapter 4 outlines the basic guidelines for planning an individualized exercise program.

The importance of stretching and warm-up cannot be emphasized enough. In Chapter 5, we provide you with a series of stretching and conditioning exercises to incorporate into your overall workout.

Making a lifetime commitment to physical fitness and wellness is one of the most important commitments you can make. The first five chapters will help you plan and structure a fitness program. This is the first step on the road to living your life to its fullest potential.

1

High-Level Health And Wellness

THE WELLNESS CONTINUUM

How is your health? Most likely you'd answer, "I'm fine." If you haven't been to a doctor or been sick recently, you would probably say that you are healthy. Most people who are able to carry out their everyday activities believe they're in good shape. In other words, they're not sick.

This concept of health is outdated. In the past, health meant only the absence of disease. Today, experts look at health in a much broader perspective. Health is a state of physical, mental, social, and emotional wellness.

Today we think of health in terms of degrees. Figure 1-1 presents the wellness continuum. It illustrates the broad scope of health from illness and early death to a high level of health.

Many people fall in the middle or neutral zone. People at this point are not ill and may look well, but they are not especially healthy either. Even though the health risks at the middle of this continuum are not fatal, living at a level of "just getting by" robs you of many opportunities. Poor health behaviors over a long time tend to be detrimental to good health in later life.

High level health means more than just getting by. It's more than going to work, attending classes, participating in organizations, and getting along with family and friends. It means having a lot of energy, eating properly, being physically active, and having a good self-concept.

Where do you place yourself on the wellness continuum? Are you living life at your fullest potential?

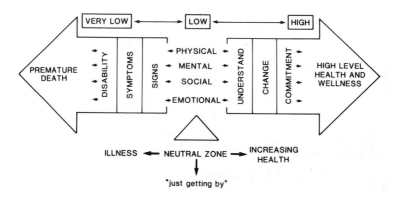

Figure 1-1. The wellness continuum.

This book focuses on how regular exercise can help you improve your health and physical fitness. Participating in a regular exercise program is a key factor in furthering good personal health.

The book includes information to help you begin and maintain an effective and enjoyable exercise program. You will learn the particulars about being properly tested. Easy-to-follow charts for walking, running, cycling, and swimming have been prepared to help you exercise at a reasonable and safe intensity. Suggestions for many more healthy exercise activities have also been included.

The simplicity of this book may surprise you. It represents a sifting of current knowledge on fitness and exercise. In fact, careful attention was given to making the book adaptable to programs with which you may be currently involved. It will reinforce any well-managed exercise program in the country.

The United States Centers for Disease Control has identified four factors that *determine* health. They include *personal health behavior, biological influences such as heredity, the conditions of your physical environment, such as air pollution and stress factors, and the quality of health care services.*

Personal health behaviors are factors in 51 percent of all major causes of death. How you behave can help you avoid serious complications in the years ahead.

Exercise is the positive "do" for helping you enjoy a healthy life. It's up to you to assume responsibility for your own health, well-being, and fitness.

WHY PHYSICAL FITNESS?

We have become a society of watchers. Not only do we sit and watch television, but we are bombarded with messages from the "electronic

Seven key factors for promoting good health are:

- Participate in regular exercise
- Sleep 7 to 8 hours a day
- Eat breakfast
- Do not eat between meals
- Maintain normal weight
- Do not smoke
- Drink in moderation

A California study by Breslow and others revealed that seven health practices were highly related with the physical health of almost 7,000 people.

authority." Advertisements promote instant cures for ailments ranging from headaches to insomnia. Promotions for soft drinks, munchies, and fast foods perpetuate poor nutritional habits. Marketing messages for energy-saving devices from riding lawn mowers to luxurious automobiles permeate prime time.

Living in a fast-paced, competitive society filled with domestic and professional obligations, we go from one demanding situation to the next. Excessive stress can damage the body. Many people seek relief through tranquilizers and alcohol, which can be detrimental to their health.

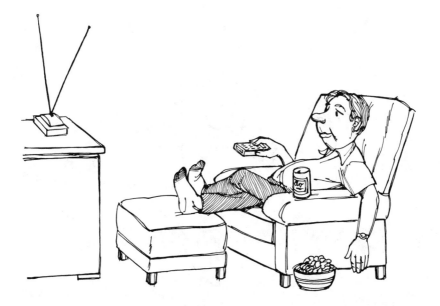

Inactivity is unhealthy. Muscles lose strength, body fat accumulates, stamina declines, the heart weakens, and blood vessels thicken. Many of these changes go undetected. We tend to accept the changes as signs of aging—not the result of inactivity.

Daily work does not provide enough exercise for health and well-being. Of course, running up and down steps or standing all day is physical exertion; however, such limited activities do not maintain fitness. You must use energy to gain energy. Regular exercise produces greater strength, endurance, and many other characteristics that come with good health. These traits can never be acquired if you sit at a desk all day, watch television, ride escalators and lawn mowers, and drive everywhere. Some authorities suggest exercise may be the cheapest preventive medicine in the world.

WHAT IS PHYSICAL FITNESS?

Being physically fit means having your heart, blood vessels, lungs, and muscles functioning at peak efficiency. You carry out your daily work and leisure activities with enthusiasm and pleasure. The five essential qualities of a physically fit body are strength, muscular endurance, flexibility, trimness, and cardiorespiratory endurance.

A sixth quality is often added—neuromuscular skill, which reflects the muscles' ability to function harmoniously and efficiently. High-level neuromuscular skill is seen in the flawless performance of experienced athletes; however, we all have the capacity to fine-tune this quality.

Although strength, muscular endurance, flexibility, and trimness

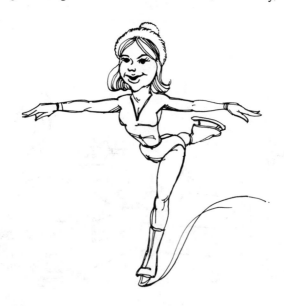

are important, **cardiorespiratory endurance** is viewed as the most essential physical fitness component. Cardiorespiratory endurance refers to the strength of your heart and lungs and your energy levels. The capacity of your heart, blood vessels, and lungs to deliver nutrients and oxygen to your tissues and to remove waste products is a key ingredient to good health and fitness. Regular, moderately intense exercise helps you develop and maintain an efficient, well-functioning cardiorespiratory system.

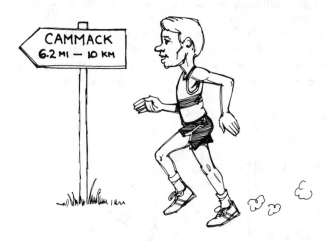

Strength, probably the most familiar component of fitness, is the capacity of a muscle to exert or resist force. Strength training results in some enlargement of the muscle fibers and a relative increase in your ability to apply force.

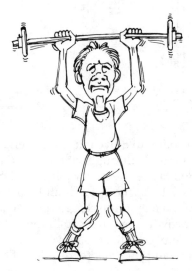

Strength is fundamental to all sports and many everyday activities. A lack of strength contributes to poor performance. Some men and many women lack upper body strength which impairs not only the ability to swing a golf club or a tennis racquet, but also the ability to mow the lawn, do housework, and carry groceries. Back pain in many adults is linked to weakness in the major abdominal muscles.

Muscular endurance is the capacity of a muscle or a group of muscles to sustain repeated contractions. It is often used incorrectly to mean strength. It also refers to the ability of a muscle to hold a fixed or static contraction over an extended period of time. In other words, muscular endurance is the ability of a muscle to apply strength and sustain it. Repeated sit-ups and push-ups test muscular endurance levels. The ability to perform everyday tasks like raking leaves, painting, and cleaning requires some degree of prolonged muscular exertion.

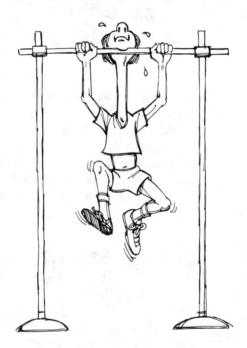

Flexibility is the ability to move joints—to bend, stretch, and twist. It's the ability to use a muscle throughout its maximum range of motion. Maintaining good mobility of the major joints of the body helps you to move about with ease. Household tasks and yard work require some degree of elasticity in the major muscle groups. Most recreational sports and physical fitness activities require a full range of muscle movement. Flexibility assures graceful coordinated movements. With increased inactivity and aging, joints and muscles tend to lose flexibility.

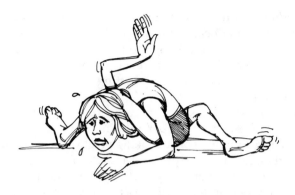

Trimness or body composition refers to the relative amounts of fat and lean body tissue (bone, muscle, and organ) that constitute your body. Relative body fat is the percentage of the total body weight that is fat.

Most experts agree that the main cause of obesity is inactivity, not overeating. Being "overfat" increases your risk for developing serious medical problems. Regular exercise is a practical approach to weight management. Fit individuals tend to burn more calories than the unfit.

How fat are you? What is your desired weight? Methods to answer these questions are presented in Chapter 12.

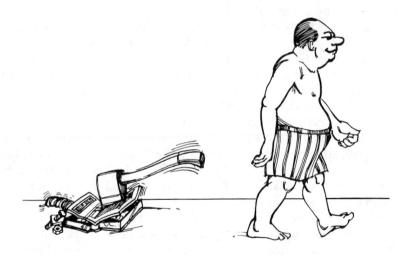

HOW EXERCISE MAKES YOU PHYSICALLY FIT

When your entire body is subjected to regular, moderately intense exercise, your general physical efficiency improves. When you are fit, your body adjusts more easily to increased physical demands. A fit heart pumps more blood per beat and beats at a lower rate at rest. Your capacity to use oxygen increases, giving you more energy to enjoy life. Although regular exercise is not a cure-all, it gives you the ability to do more and feel better when doing it. Getting more out of life is the best reward of being fit!

If you follow this book's basic guidelines, you will gain a better understanding of exercise's proper role in your life. Once exercise is incorporated into your life, you are taking positive steps toward reaching a safe and attainable level of physical fitness. Your goal—to sustain a moderately-intense endurance-type activity at an effort level of between 60 and 80 percent of your maximal capacity for a minimum of 30 minutes at least four times a week. You probably won't attain this goal within the first few weeks of a personalized exercise program. That's okay. Our step-by-step exercise charts will make it easier for you to exercise within your capabilities on a regular basis. Eventually you will become physically fit.

MAKING THE COMMITMENT

Whatever your reason for starting an exercise program you must make a firm pledge to stay with it. This commitment is paramount, especially during the initial weeks.

As a rule, it takes at least three to four months for most people to fully appreciate the pleasures of stimulating exercise. You have to stay with it long enough to reap the rewards. When you reach this point, you will likely be working out not because you have to, but because you want to. You will not only be thinking fitness and health, but you will be practicing fitness and health.

Can you handle such a commitment? The answer is yes. Daily living takes some planning and discipline; reporting to work, caring for families, keeping appointments, and meeting deadlines are already essential parts of your demanding lifestyle. Becoming physically fit and maintaining fitness will become additional commitments. It all comes back to the question of your priorities. Living at optimal physiological health has to be a priority. It warrants the investments of time and effort.

There are 168 hours in the week. All you need is about four 30-minute workouts of sustained exercise per week and four 15-minute sessions of strength and muscular endurance workouts to attain and maintain a reasonable fitness level. Add at least another 15 minutes to each workout for warming up and cooling down. Figure 30 minutes for dressing and showering before and after your workout. That's a total of six hours a week for better health and fitness. This is a small investment of time and effort for such a large and beneficial return.

Getting Started

You can never begin too low (in the exercise charts), and the progressive steps you take can never be too small. Injuries and discouragement result when you try to make up in a few weeks what you lost over years of sedentary living.

Do not try to change everything at once. A regular exercise program usually provides incentive to change such debilitating habits as smoking, excessive drinking, and overeating. But start by getting into shape. Then you can more effectively tackle poor habits. People who undertake an exercise program and try to quit smoking or make drastic nutritional changes all at once generally fail.

Staying With It

We all encounter stumbling blocks when we try to fit everything— including regular exercise—into our schedules. Lack of time, illness (and not necessarily your own), family obligations, laziness (we all experience this), bad weather, and injuries can easily sidetrack a well-intended fitness endeavor. Such conflicts can be disconcerting, and for some people, reason enough to quit. Here are suggestions on how to overcome these obstacles.

Finding time to exercise can be difficult unless you know where to look for it. Honestly appraise your day. Examine your calendar and take a good look at your activities to find a time that is best for your schedule.

Setting aside a specific time of the day for exercise increases your chances of working out on a regular basis. It's easy to say "I'll do it tonight," and then when evening comes, "I'll do it in the morning." Set a definite time best for you and stick to it. See whether your company has a morning, noontime, or after work exercise program. Many adults find early morning is an excellent time for working out while others tend to favor noon hours. Even though occasional adjustments are inevitable, setting a specific time for exercise lessens the chances of failure.

Another tactic is to workout with your spouse, friends or work colleagues. Working out with others provides a stimulus to keep you going. Group programs, found at many YMCAs, YWCAs, community centers, and corporate and private fitness centers provide opportunities to meet other fitness enthusiasts. Many corporations and businesses are developing exercise programs as part of health promotion for their employees.

Do not overlook the value of keeping a daily record of your workouts. It not only provides a progress report, but also monitors your weekly efforts. The progressive workout charts presented later in this book will help those of you starting out. A record is most helpful during the early weeks of training. It actually becomes fun to note when you exercise, how long you exercise, how far you went, and how you felt.

Many private and corporate workout centers now have computerized check-in and check-out stations. Experience indicates people who do not keep records tend to be very sporadic and do not adhere to a regular exercise program.

A well-planned exercise workout strengthens your chances for improvement. Don't expect to see instant results. Successful improvement in physical fitness comes in spurts. Every day will not be glorious. Each workout will not result in euphoria. However, the progressive workout charts in the latter sections of the book are set up to guide you through the good and bad days. Each step is designed so you can complete it without becoming overly fatigued, but still get the necessary stimulation for your heart, lungs, and muscles.

You may feel some discomfort when you exercise. This feeling will vary from day to day and from person to person. Remember, if you are quite uncomfortable and exhausted an hour after you exercise, you are probably overdoing it. Adjust your next workout. The aim of this book is to show you how to keep your workouts reasonably comfortable, to avoid unnecessary fatigue, and to help you develop your fitness potential.

The strongest reinforcement for staying with a regular exercise program is simply how you feel. After a few weeks you'll feel stronger, more alert, and more relaxed than you did when you started. One of the main reasons people stay with an exercise program is they *really* do feel better. Although feeling good is reason enough, taking off fat and maintaining a stronger heart and circulatory system are the bonuses of a more active lifestyle.

2

Know Your Body

Your body is meant to be used. Before embarking on a fitness program it helps if you understand how exercise nourishes the body. This chapter will provide you with an overview of how your body functions, responds to exercise, and becomes stronger and more efficient with proper exercise.

HEART AND LUNGS

Your heart, lungs, blood, and various muscle cells are interdependent parts making up the cardiorespiratory system. Each cell needs a ready supply of oxygen and food for energy and the means by which to rid itself of carbon dioxide and other waste products. Your circulatory and respiratory systems work together to provide these services. Because of their interdependence, the two systems are referred to as the cardiorespiratory system. A moderately intensive rhythmic exercise program is the key to keeping your cardiorespiratory system functioning efficiently.

The Heart

Your heart beats constantly, pumping blood throughout your body at approximately 72 beats per minutes or more than 100,000 beats in 24 hours. It is capable of circulating at least 2,000 gallons of blood a day.

This muscle, a little larger than your fist, is composed of two upper chambers called atria and two lower chambers called ventricles (Figure 2-1). The right atrium and the right ventricle are separated from their counterparts on the left by a muscular wall. This separation wall allows the heart to work as two separate pumps (right and left).

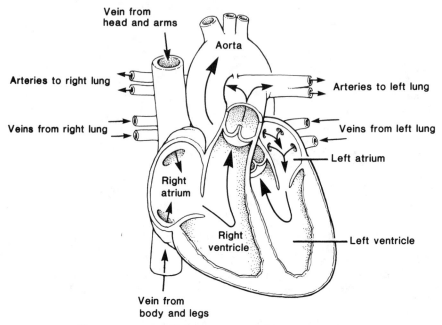

Figure 2-1. Cross-section of the heart.

Each atrium is connected to its corresponding ventricle by a one-way valve. The right atrium receives blood, low in oxygen, from the body and pumps it through the right ventricle to the lungs. At the same time, the left atrium receives fresh, oxygen-rich blood from the lungs and pumps it through the left ventricle and out the aorta, your body's largest artery, to all the body's tissues.

The blood passing through the chambers of the heart does not nourish the heart muscle. Instead, arterial branches called coronary arteries, which originate from the aorta, direct blood through numerous branches over the outer surface of the heart (Figure 2-2). These branches, embedded in the muscle tissues of the heart, divide into smaller arteries and capillaries in the heart muscle. In this way each cardiac muscle fiber receives constant nourishment. The blood is then returned to the right atrium through the coronary sinus, a large vein formed by the coronary veins.

The Lungs

The lungs, located within the rib cage, regulate the exchange of air between the blood and the external environment (Figure 2-3). After air enters the body through the nose or mouth, it passes into the throat which branches into two tubes, the esophagus, where food passes to the stomach, and the trachea, the air passage.

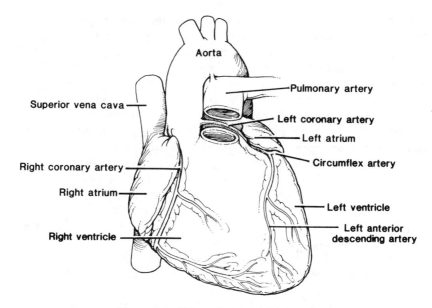

Figure 2-2. External view of the heart.

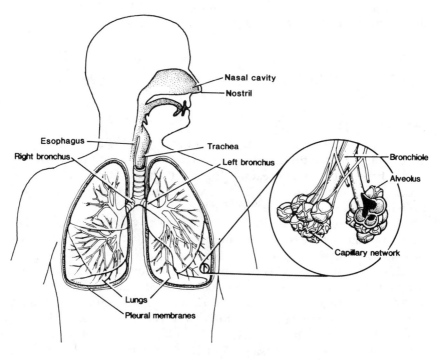

Figure 2-3. The lungs.

The trachea extends downward toward the lungs. It divides into two branches called bronchi, one leading to each lung. Within each lung each brochus divides and subdivides throughout the entire organ. Eventually this subdivision ends in tiny ducts attached to an estimated one billion microscopic air sacs called alveoli. These clustered-together air sacs give the lungs their spongy texture. Blood capillaries surround the alveoli.

When air is breathed into the lungs, oxygen molecules pass through the walls of the air sacs into the capillaries. Here in the capillaries they combine with molecules of hemoglobin, the protein-iron pigment in the red blood cells. From the lungs, this oxygenated blood returns to the left side of the heart where it is pumped to all parts of the body. Throughout the body, oxygen is picked up by the cells, and in turn, the blood picks up carbon dioxide and other waste products. Carbon dioxide is returned through the veins to the heart and then to the lungs where it is eventually breathed out through the nose and mouth.

At rest the lungs breathe in about six to eight liters (one liter equals 1.06 quarts) of air each minute. This rate increases during the mildest exertion.

When you walk, climb stairs, or exercise, your cells require more oxygen. Breathing increases in both depth and rate according to the intensity and duration of the exertion.

The level of ventilation may reach well over 100 liters a minute in an all-out athletic performance.

CARDIORESPIRATORY RESPONSES

The Heart Rate

The heart rate, (the number of beats per minute) and the amount of blood pumped from the heart with each beat, varies with the changing needs of the body. When resting, the heart pumps about five liters of blood a minute, but it is capable of increasing this cardiac output to 15 to 25 liters of blood a minute when the body is active.

Your resting heart rate (RHR) is influenced by your age, your level of cardiorespiratory fitness, and environmental factors. It tends to become lower as your fitness improves.

Resting heart rates vary from extremes of below 40 beats per minute in highly trained athletes to over 100 beats per minute in sedentary adults. The average for most adults is 72 beats per minute. Women tend to have higher sitting heart rates than men. People who exercise regularly often have rates between 50 to 60 beats per minute or lower.

When you begin exercising, your heart rate increases. During low levels of exercise sustained over a period of time, your elevated heart rate will level out at a constant rate. The increase in heart rate during exercise is directly proportional to the intensity of the exercise.

An example of this is shown in Figure 2-4. Notice how the subject's heart rate increased as the walking speed on the treadmill test increased from 3.0 mph to a brisker pace of 3.5 mph (a 17-minute-per-mile speed). At the four-minute mark the heart rate of this 40-year-old man was 136 beats per minute. (He had been leading a sedentary life prior to this test.) After four minutes of level walking, the treadmill incline was raised to 4 percent and every two minutes thereafter, increased 2 percent. Note how the heart rate increased as his body responded to the increased demands at each grade of the walking task.

The increase in heart rate is in direct proportion to the increase in workload, up to a limit. As his exercise workload became more difficult, he eventually reached the stage of the test where he began to peak and eventually had to stop (at 8 percent grade and at the nine-minute mark). At this point his heart rate reached 183 beats per minute, representing his highest attainable maximal heart rate. When you perform strenuous exercise to exhaustion, the heart rate at this point is your *maximal or peak heart rate.*

In Chapter 4 you will learn how to regulate the intensity of a workout using your heart rate. Knowing your maximal heart rate helps you determine your training or target heart rate. You can estimate your maximal heart rate based on your age or you can have it tested, as explained in Chapter 3.

Maximal heart rates of 180 to 200 beats per minute are quite common. Your maximal heart rate declines with age. It has little relationship

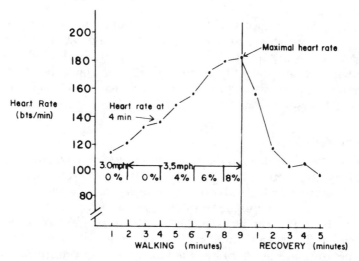

Figure 2-4. Heart rate response on a treadmill.

to your state of fitness and can generally be estimated to be close to 220 minus your age. As you can see, applying this rule for estimating the 40-year-old man's maximal heart rate comes pretty close to his actual maximal rate (220 - 40 = 180).

At any given heart rate, a heart with a larger capacity per beat (a larger stroke volume) will pump more blood. It has a higher cardiac output for the same heart rate. (Stroke volume times heart rate equals cardiac output.) The larger the stroke volume, the greater the heart's ability to pump blood, and the higher the level of its performance.

Heart rate responses to standardized exercise tests (testings utilizing the same working rate) are convenient indicators of circulatory efficiency and fitness. Figure 2-5 shows the heart rate data for a 55-year-old man. His heart rate was monitored while he walked for nine minutes on a treadmill. He was tested before beginning a run-walk exercise program and again after 10 weeks of training four days a week. He was able to run a little over a mile without stopping when he was tested at the 10-week point. At this time his heart's response for the same walking task clearly shows a more efficient circulatory response. His heart rate at each minute of walking was decidedly lower throughout the walking test than it was prior to training. His heart was pumping the same amount of blood more efficiently at a lower heart rate and a higher stroke volume.

To further illustrate the effects of training on the heart, he was tested one year later performing the same walking task. At this time, he was running four times a week and averaging three miles each workout. Notice the lower heart rate throughout each minute of the walking test. At the last minute of exercise the graph clearly shows a drop from 133 (beginning of the program) to 124 (after 10 weeks) to 110 after a year of regular exercise.

A more rapid recovery of the heart rate to its resting level after a workout also indicates cardiac efficiency. Again look at Figure 2-5 and notice how the man's heart recovered faster after 10 weeks and one year of training. The physically fit person generally has a lower heart rate and a more rapid recovery time for any given exercise workload. In other words, a fit person is a healthier person.

Blood Pressure

Blood pressure refers to the amount of pressure maintained in your arteries by the pumping action of your heart and the resistance of your blood vessels to blood flow. Blood pressure is generally recorded as two numbers. The higher number (systolic pressure) reflects the force the blood exerts against the walls of the vessels as the heart contracts and ejects blood. The lower number (diastolic pressure) measures the reduced pressure in the arteries as the blood flows toward the veins and the heart relaxes and refills.

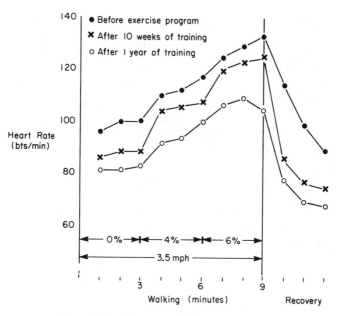

Figure 2-5. Heart rate changes in training.

While sitting, the systolic pressure in a normal, healthy person is approximately 120 millimeters (mm) and the diastolic pressure is around 80 mm, expressed $^{120}\!/_{80}$ mm Hg. Hypertension means high arterial pressure or simply "high blood pressure." A resting pressure of $^{140}\!/_{90}$ mm Hg or higher is generally considered high blood pressure.

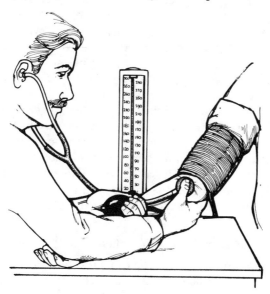

The causes of high blood pressure are often unknown. However, we know high blood pressure places an abnormal strain on the heart and arteries and is a primary risk factor for heart disease. Therefore, many doctors feel even a mild case of hypertension warrants attention.

Medication and controlling diet and the level of salt intake help to keep the blood pressure within normal limits. Furthermore, rhythmic, moderately intense, endurance-type exercises such as running, swimming, cycling, and brisk walking are sound means for lowering the resting blood pressure and keeping it down.

During exercise, the systolic pressure increases, primarily because of increases in cardiac output. This rise in blood pressure is a normal response to the intensity of the activities. Researchers believe this higher systolic pressure and the resulting dilation of the arteries during exercise tend to benefit the blood-flow mechanisms and help keep the resting blood pressure at normal levels.

Lung Function

When you exercise your cells need more oxygen. Your body's demand for more oxygen is met by an increased breathing and blood flow. The ability to improve your capacity to breathe more air and to transport oxygen more rapidly to the cells are key factors in developing a healthy and fit body.

During vigorous exercise, the body's inability to get enough oxygen and the metabolic build-up of waste products hinder the muscles' ability to contract. Your movements become impaired. Your lungs always contain ample oxygen for the circulating blood to pick up as it passes through them. Furthermore, the oxygenated blood leaving the lungs and returning to the heart is almost always saturated with oxygen. The problem, therefore, is to get more blood to the active muscle tissues to meet the needs of exertion. These needs can be met by increasing the speed with which the blood goes through the cardiovascular system.

The key to successful muscular performance is the heart's ability to pump blood and the muscles' ability to use the oxygen. Your exercise performance, then, is limited to the highest levels at which your heart, lungs, and blood vessels can function. When you feel "out of breath" or become exhausted during even mild exercise, it is not due to a shortage of oxygen in the lungs. Instead, it is due to your heart's inability to pump sufficient blood to the muscle tissues as well as your cells' failure to receive adequate amounts of oxygen to meet the energy needs.

Aerobic Capacity (Maximal Oxygen Uptake)

The largest amount of oxygen you can consume per minute is called your maximal oxygen uptake (VO2 max). This maximal value, often referred to as maximal aerobic capacity, is the functional measure of physical fitness. Your body's capacity to sustain effort over a prolonged period of time is limited by the blood's ability to deliver oxygen to your active tissues. Theoretically, a higher oxygen uptake indicates the increased ability of 1) the heart to pump blood, 2) the lungs to ventilate larger volumes of air, and 3) the muscle cells to take up oxygen and remove carbon dioxide.

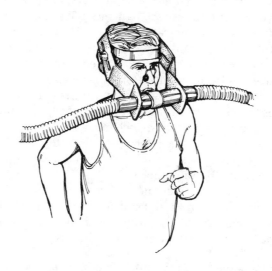

Not all of us can improve our maximal oxygen uptakes to the same extent, even with similar types of training. Each person seems to have a certain genetically-determined potential for optimal development. The physical characteristics of parents predispose some individuals to adapt more favorably to training than others. While regular vigorous exercise can increase your maximal aerobic capacity by as much as 20 to 30 percent, the precise amount of improvement depends on your genetic endowment, initial fitness level, and the intensity and duration of your exercise program.

GENDER CONSIDERATIONS

Research suggests that the way both sexes respond to vigorous physical activity is much more similar than different. Although women have lower values for maximal oxygen uptake, their rates of improvement are similar to those of men. Women's exercise heart rates tend to also improve proportionately with those of the men. When differences in body size and structure are taken into account, women's responses to vigorous exercise are essentially the same as men's.

Studies of sedentary middle-age and older women and men have repeatedly shown that although women had lower values of maximal oxygen uptake, their rates of improvement with exercise were similar to those of men. Exercise heart rates also improved (that is decreased) proportionately with those of the men. Loss of skinfold fat at selected sites was also comparable.

There is no scientific evidence to substantiate the notion that vigorous exercise will make women appear excessively muscular. Women normally have less muscle mass than men. The inherent capacity for muscle development is genetically determined by the sex hormone levels. The male hormone, testosterone, is responsible for muscle bulkiness in men. This hormone is present in women, but in amounts probably too low to have a substantial effect on muscle size.

However, the development of muscle mass is as varied among women as it is among men. Women in general have less muscle mass (23 percent compared to 40 percent muscle mass of a man's body), a lighter bone structure, and more body fat. Therefore, for people of the same height, a woman will usually weigh less than a man, and she will have less power to propel the same mass.

To date, no laboratory evidence exists to substantiate recent claims that women naturally burn more fat as muscle fuel and perhaps may be better suited to endurance performance than men. However, we do know that endurance training does assist the working muscles to make efficient use of fat for energy.

Women generally have less muscle mass, fewer total red blood cells and about 15 percent less hemoglobin (the protein-iron molecule that carries oxygen in the blood) than men. Consequently, a woman cannot carry as much oxygen in her blood as a man, a factor that may limit her endurance.

AGE CONSIDERATIONS

In recent years there have been several major studies on exercise and the aging. In 1986, Ralph S. Paffenbarger, M.D., of the Stanford University School of Medicine, concluded Americans can lead longer lives if they engage in ongoing physical exercise. His research shows we lessen our chances of early death if we increase our levels of physical activity. Rather than suffering prolonged periods of declining health, regular exercisers tend to enjoy active old age with rapid declines at the end.

Dr. Everett Smith, University of Wisconsin, has been involved with developing exercise programs for the older adult. From his experiences he feels strongly that age should not be a limiting factor for anyone wishing to participate in physical activity. In fact, he feels physical ac-

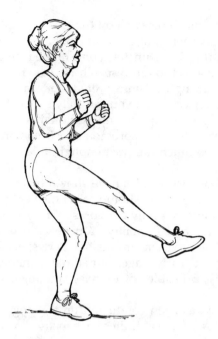

tivity is important for older adults in maintaining good health and well-being. Research studies indicate that as much as 50 percent of physiological decline is related to disuse and that a high level of physiological function can be maintained into the later years of aging with regular physical activity.

To our way of thinking, as you get older, you need to exercise more, but perhaps at a lesser intensity. The less vigorous your exercise, the more important it is to exercise a little longer each session and on a more regular basis.

THE BENEFITS OF EXERCISE

Now that you have a clearer understanding of how your body works and responds to exercise, it is time to consider the benefits of exercise.

A plethora of information exists proclaiming the benefits of exercise. Much of it goes too far. Enthusiastic promoters often make false claims or statements having no scientific backing. Programs promising total fitness in 30 minutes a week or thin thighs in 30 days unfortunately sell lots of books but fail to produce the promised results. This section describes the proven beneficial effects of regular exercise.

Regardless of your age, rhythmic endurance-type exercise (practiced according to the guidelines in Chapter 4) can yield predictable, beneficial effects. The extent of these positive changes varies from person to person.

In recent years, much research on the effects of exercise training on the human body has been conducted in laboratories and fitness centers throughout the world. Unfortunately some of the results never reach the general public. Worse yet, often research results are twisted, taken out of context, or unknowingly misinterpreted. For example, manufacturers of weight-training devices claim you can fully develop cardiorespiratory fitness just by using their equipment. Although scientific studies have refuted such statements, these promoters artfully cite research, being careful not to say too much, but just enough to lead consumers to buy their equipment.

Controlled laboratory studies have shown that some forms of exercise are better than others. You should select the best activities for developing and maintaining not only cardiorespiratory fitness but strength, muscular endurance, and flexibility. You need to develop a safe and reasonable plan. The programs in this book are specifically designed to guide you through the early stages of getting in shape. These plans are based on the latest principles of exercise training and valid scientific studies.

Much research has been conducted on walking, running, cycling, and swimming. Most of these studies have focused on training regimens that progressively increase exercise workload as improvement occurs. The researchers have been concerned with how the body adapts to varying intensities of exercise within the tolerance level of the participants.

In Chapter 4 we will show you how the basic information derived from research studies can be applied to help you plan your fitness workouts. No matter whether you walk, run, swim, or cycle, you will be in a scientifically-tested program.

Improved Heart Functions

After eight to 10 weeks of vigorous endurance-type exercise performed on a regular basis (four times a week), your heart begins to beat less, not only at rest, but during everyday tasks. Your heart will be working more efficiently, pumping more blood with fewer strokes. Furthermore, it will recover more rapidly from any type of activity.

The cumulative effect of a drop in the number of heart beats over a 24-hour period is impressive. Let's say, as a result of exercise training, you reduce your average heart rate by 10 beats (a common occurrence) for each minute of the day. That means you will save about 14,400 beats per day. This improved pumping efficiency allows the heart to work more effectively both at rest and during physical exertion. Some people in research studies have reduced their resting heart rates by as much as 15 or more beats per minute.

The heart rates of fit individuals increase less during standard exercise tests than do those of inactive persons. Figure 2-6 presents information about a group of eight previously inactive women who exercised using the methods presented in this book. As they progressed, they were tested for nine minutes at a moderate walking speed of 3 mph, or a 20-minute-mile pace. This type of test is referred to as a submaximal test. Most people (whether they exercise or not) should be able to complete it.

Notice how the average heart rate for these women (average age 38) is lowered as they progress through 20 weeks of rhythmic endurance-type exercise. Throughout each minute of this moderate exercise test improvement occurred. In the last (ninth) minute they averaged a heart rate of 131 prior to the exercise program. Ten weeks later the ninth-minute heart rate was down to 124, and after 20 weeks of walking and running it was at 118—a 13-beat reduction.

Improved Oxygen Uptake

During exercise the muscle tissues develop mechanisms to use greater volumes of oxygen. These adaptations, which readily result from endurance-type training, are determined by measuring one's maximal oxygen uptake capacity.

Because a larger person with more muscle mass has the capability to use more oxygen than the smaller person, aerobic capacity (maximal oxygen uptake) is expressed in relation to body weight (ml/kg min or milliliters of oxygen per kilogram of weight per minute.) Young college-age males and females range between values of 42 to 44 and 38 to 41 ml/kg min, respectively. Older people and people who have lead sedentary lives tend to show lower values. For a sedentary 40-year-old man, aero-

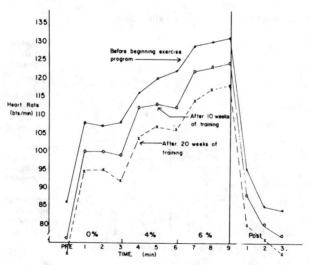

Figure 2-6. Comparative heart rate changes in training.

bic capacity can drop to 30 to 34 ml/kg min. Fortunately, exercise studies repeatedly show that the decline in aerobic capacity as one ages can be slowed and even improved to the point where an older person's aerobic fitness can be higher than the average for young people.

Figure 2-7 summarizes the effects of different modes of training on maximal oxygen uptake. Notice the levels of maximal oxygen uptake before training and the relative change over periods ranging from 10 to 15 weeks.

Blood Pressure Changes

Several studies have indicated that active people tend to have lower resting blood pressures than most sedentary people. If your blood pressure is normal, vigorous endurance-type exercise has little, if any, effect on blood pressure. Some people with high blood pressure may see dramatic changes to more normal levels with exercise.

To claim exercise alone lowers blood pressure is still debatable. For people who already have serious complications related to high blood pressure, the benefits of exercise may be limited. The combination of an altered diet, medication, and exercise appears to be a promising approach to controlling this major risk factor of heart disease.

Improved Blood Lipid Levels

In your blood right now are various kinds of particles carrying fat around to do important work or get stored for later use. One of those substances is cholesterol, a substance produced in the liver. It is essential

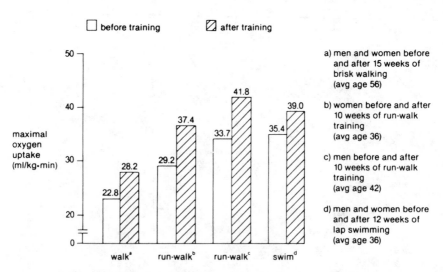

Figure 2-7. Training modes and maximal oxygen uptakes.

for cell structure and for the formation of various hormones, including sex hormones. Cholesterol and fatty substances called triglycerides also make up the atherosclerotic deposits on the inner lining of the arteries that eventually may lead to heart disease. Medical researchers believe cholesterol floating in the blood is in part the source of this continual accumulation.

Cholesterol levels can be measured and are expressed in milligrams per deciliter (100 milliters) of blood. Any value above 250 mg/dl is considered dangerous. What is normal? The National Institutes of Health recommends keeping your blood cholesterol level below 200 mg/dl. Experts believe that consuming diets high in animal fat and cholesterol and leading inactive lifestyles are both related to high cholesterol levels in some people.

The fat particles called triglycerides represesnt 95 percent of all fats stored in the body. When more calories are eaten than are used for energy, the excess is turned into triglycerides (fat), transported in the blood, and stored in fat cells situated throughout the body (abdomen, thighs, arms, and chin). These fats also seem to be related to atherosclerosis and, like cholesterol, can be lowered by weight loss through dieting and exercise. Research experts have shown dramatic drops of triglyeride levels with aerobic exercise.

Cholesterol is carried in the bloodstream by certain proteins, called lipoproteins, because they carry lipids (fats). Three types of lipoprotein are especially important to heart disease: high-density lipoprotein (HDL), low-density lipoprotein (LDL), and very-low-density lipoprotein (VLDL). The VLDLs transport triglycerides from the liver to the fat cells for storage throughout the body. The LDLs carry cholesterol from the liver to the cells of various tissues where it is used to make cell membranes and certain hormones. And the HDLs, the "good" lipoprotein, clear the unneeded cholesterol from the tissues and return it to the liver for excretion.

For years the medical profession has known the cholesterol being deposited in the arteries (atherosclerosis) is the cholesterol attached to the low-density lipoprotein (LDL). Although the role of HDLs is not clearly understood, they are thought to prevent cholesterol from sticking to the inner walls of the arteries, thereby thwarting the process of atherosclerosis. In other words, people with high levels of HDL cholesterol in the blood tend to be relatively free of heart disease, whereas those with high LDL levels are more likely to suffer heart attacks.

Current research suggests that active people can raise their HDL levels and presumably move toward a more favorable risk category; however, it remains to be demonstrated how much activity and at what intensity these measures are affected. Weight loss and low-fat diets also seem be important in bringing about improvements.

Exercising offers no guarantee you will live longer than your sedentary friends, but you are likely to live closer to your full genetic potential. A well-organized, vigorous physical fitness program should focus on adding more life to your years. Adding more years to your life may be the bonus.

Weight Management

Many people doubt the effectiveness of exercise as a means for weight loss. The National Institute firmly believes that, for most people, being overweight is a problem of being inactive. Body weight can be controlled by engaging regularly in moderately intense exercise.

As we age, activity levels tend to decrease, while appetites and eating habits do not. In fact, appetite may even increase. Calories that are consumed but not used are usually stored as fat.

Contrary to what some so-called diet experts say, cutting back on calories alone does not enable a person to have a lean and healthy appearance. In fact, we can emphatically say exercise is the key ingredient in taking off excess fat. Exercise must be part of your weight management plan, or you will still look flabby.

Research shows exercise or exercise with a modified diet is better for weight reduction than dieting alone. People who exercise reflect in-

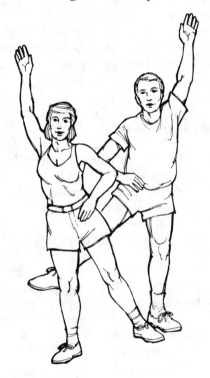

creases in lean muscle tissue as well as losses of fat. However, during the early stages of training, as the muscle mass increases and fat burns off, the scales often remain the same, which to the uninformed, becomes discouraging. In contrast, many special diets (such as low-carbohydrates diets) often result in rapid fluid loss and, in some cases, even loss of muscle tissue, leading to the false belief that fat has been lost. Usually, as soon as the dieter returns to a normal diet, they regain the water and the weight comes back. Weight management is covered more fully in Chapter 12.

Lean body tissue represents the bone-muscle-organ tissue of your body. This part of your body, often called fat-free tissue, gives the body its shape. Rhythmic moderately-intense exercise builds up firm and supple muscles.

As your muscles become stronger, they increase somewhat in size. However, these continuous and rhythmical activities do not make bulky muscles. And in women, this increase in muscle fiber thickness is not as great as in men. With the expected fat loss, your girths, if abnormally large to start with, will actually become smaller despite this muscle development.

Psychological Effects

Recent reviews and historical evidence on the psychological effects of exercise strongly suggest an association between exercise and an improved state of mind. The Greeks wrote of *mena sana in corpore sans;* translated, that means "a healthy mind in a healthy body."

Being physically fit bolsters your self-image and helps you to be more positive about those around you. Besides providing a diversion from the everyday work, engaging in exercise provides excellent mental relief and relaxation. Exercise builds a body that performs better at everything one does during the day.

Kenneth Cooper, M.D., founder and director of The Aerobics Institute in Dallas, Texas, believes physically-fit people tend to be psychologically fit. They exhibit a "fitness glow." They feel better, look better, and have an improved self-image. "When people become physically fit, they feel better because they are more relaxed, more in tune, more aware, and more perceptive," Cooper says.

Other research studies have attempted to explain the "high" often reported by exercisers. Although hard evidence for such a "high" isn't conclusive, the number of people who testify to such feelings is impressive. One study was conducted at Boston's Massachusetts General Hospital. A small group of women who spent two months bicycling and jogging experienced dramatic beta endorphin increases in their blood. Endorphin, an opium-like substance produced by the brain and pituitary gland, helps the body resist pain. The researchers attribute this increased release of these opium-like secretions as a possible explanation of "runners' high."

Exercise is one of the very best ways to manage chronic or excessive stress. Stress is a part of daily life. Considerable scientific literature now suggests that emotional stress has a role in the development of coronary artery disease. Emotional stress is strongly related to elevated blood cholesterol, high blood pressure, and cigarette smoking. Although strenuous exercise is a stressor, it can be very effective in tempering the harmful effects of emotional stress.

WHAT ABOUT SMOKING?

As mentioned earlier, exercise along with weight loss, may reduce higher than normal blood pressure. Although exercise won't cancel the effects of cigarette smoking, many smokers who have adhered to the exercise guidelines in this book have succeeded in giving up the addiction. A smoker pursuing a disciplined exercise program may have the best method of kicking the habit.

Let's be frank! Cigarette smoking is harmful to your health. The World Health Organization states:

"Smoking-related disease are such important causes of disability and premature death in developed countries that the control of cigarette smoking could do more to improve health and prolong life in these countries than any single action in the whole field of preventive medicine."

According to cardiologist John W. Farquhar, M.D., of the Stanford Medical School, cigarettes contribute much more to the incidence of heart attacks than to lung cancer. In fact, with other risk factors being equal, the average smoker is more than twice as likely to have a heart attack than the non-smoker.

If you are a smoker, and adhere to the program guidelines in this book, you will quickly learn that edurance-type exercise and smoking do not mix. First concentrate on the beginning stages of getting in shape. Follow the charts. Eventually, as you adjust to the early workouts and experience the positive effects of training, you will realize that smoking hinders your progress. Then you can begin to confront your smoking problem.

A key reason to quit smoking is to reduce the risk of coronary heart disease. Also, the risk of cancer is greatly reduced. Other possible benefits range from improved sleep to keener taste and smell.

SUMMARY

Now you understand why your body needs regular exercise. You are aware of changes to look for as you begin to follow the programs recommended in this book. The rest of this book provides the necessary know-how to help you realize the true benefits of exercise. Chapter 3 explains the importance of fitness testing, while Chapter 4 discusses the fundamentals of designing your own program and answers such questions as how hard, how long, and how often you have to work out. It also presents the best activities for improving cardiorespiratory fitness.

We're confident that if you carefully adhere to these recommendations, you'll discover new energies and the good feeling of being physically fit.

3

How Fit Are You?

If you have been inactive, or if you have any doubt about your state of health, getting tested before beginning an exercise program can help you understand your current fitness status and determine a safe starting point. Even if you've been exercising on a regular basis, you will find it interesting and helpful to know your fitness level in relation to other people.

Knowledge of your fitness strengths and weaknesses will enable you to set up a personalized, safe, and enjoyable exercise program. In the chapters to follow, you will find specific guidelines for developing progressive exercise workouts that allow you to stay well within your capabilities. Working out too intensely can cause discomfort and unnecessary injuries. Later when you repeat some of the tests, you will be able to gauge the effectiveness of a regular exercise program.

Exercise tests carried out to evaluate your physical fitness status are termed functional fitness tests; tests conducted to check out symptoms are termed diagnostic tests and generally carried out in a medical clinic.

Dr. P.O. Astrand, a world-renowned exercise physiologist and director of the Institute of Work Physiology in Stockholm, says this about medical examinations: "The question is frequently raised whether a medical examination is advisable before commencing a training program. Certainly, anyone doubtful about his (or her) state of health should consult a physician . . . (however) in principle, there is less risk in activity than continuous inactivity, and . . . it is more advisable to pass a careful medical examination if one intends to be sedentary (inactive) in order to establish whether one's state of health is good enough to stand the inactivity."

In fact, it would be a good decision for you to first visit your family physician for a regular checkup. Such a visit will identify any factors that might affect how you begin your personalized exercise program. Most likely you will be cleared to join an organized program or begin exercising on your own. Your physician may even suggest you get tested. Most fitness testing centers have one or more physicians associated with their programs. However, be sure to check out the expertise of any non-medical people who are going to test you. You may want to find out which centers are staffed with professionals who have undertaken the rigorous written and practical exams in testing and exercise leadership given by the American College of Sports Medicine (ACSM).

ACSM is a multi-disciplinary professional and scientific society dedicated to the generation and dissemination of information concerning the motivation, responses, and adaptations of people engaged in exercises. Its publication, *Guidelines for Graded Exercise Testing and Exercise Prescription* (Third Edition, 1986), includes current recommendations on health screening and exercise testing. According to ACSM, exercise is safe for most people. However, the college suggests that those who want to begin an exercise program be screened and take some selected exercise tests. One's age, current health status, and present activity level are factors that determine the depth of evaluation required and need for medical involvement.

ACSM has categorized individuals who undergo exercise testing:

1. Apparently healthy—those who seem to be in good health and have no major coronary heart disease risk factors.
2. Individuals at high risk—those who have one or more symptoms suggestive of possible coronary heart disease.
3. Individuals with disease—those with known heart, lung, or metabolic disease.

Evaluation or screening prior to testing helps the testing team determine your category. Screening generally includes the following components:

- Medical/health history—family history, past health, medications, smoking history, lifestyle, and activity patterns.
- Resting Physical Exam—body weight and composition (% fat), heart rate, and blood pressure.
- Selected Laboratory Tests—blood tests such as total cholesterol, high density lipoproteins, triglycerides, glucose, and others.

The medical/health history, along with a blood pressure test, are minimal requirements before you begin any type of exercise testing or exercise program.

This preliminary background information not only helps determine the proper exercise test protocol but also provides valuable information for interpreting any additional exercise tests.

If you have a known coronary heart disease or other major health problems, you *must have* the approval of a physician before you engage in any fitness testing or exercise program. Those of you with any primary risk factors for coronary heart disease or other problems (such as diabetes) need to be tested in a carefully supervised setting.

GENERAL PRINCIPLES FOR EXERCISE TESTS

Treadmill walking and/or running and stationary cycling on an ergometer are the two main modes for testing fitness. Treadmill testing is the most popular because of the ease with which both speed and elevation can be varied. The treadmill also provides for an accurate range of exercise intensities with excellent reproducibility for follow-up testing. The disadvantage of stationary cycle is that early leg fatique can slow down individuals unaccustomed to cycling before they reach their maximal heart rates.

Whether you are tested on a bicycle ergomter or a treadmill, basic principles apply to all exercise tests in a laboratory setting.

1. You will begin exercising at a low level of exertion.
2. The workload is increased gradually in two- to three-minute stages.
3. Heart rate and other measures are monitored regularly throughout the test.
4. When the exercise test is completed, all observations (heart rate, electrocardiogram) are continued for a five- to 10-minute recov-

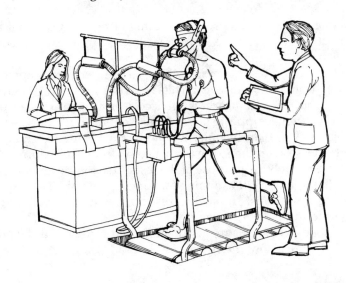

ery period unless abnormal responses occur, requiring longer post-test observations.

What to Expect

Before taking a graded exercise test (often referred to as a GXT), you'll be asked to read and sign an informed consent. This form explains the testing procedures and potential risks along with the discomforts you may feel as you are tested.

It is customary to fill out a medical-health history form before taking the GXT. Your physical activity and smoking patterns are noted, and questions may be asked about your nutritional habits, recent body weight changes, and stress in your everyday life. All information is held in confidence.

During the non-activity portion of the test, a resting 12-lead electrocardiogram (ECG) is administered. A resting ECG is not likely to detect any abnormalities unless you have advanced coronary heart disease. Nevertheless, a resting record may be helpful in later years as a reference if changes do occur. Your resting blood pressure and heart rate are routinely measured. Usually height, weight, and body fat measurements are also taken. A blood draw is often a part of pre-test procedures. The key blood measures affected by exercise and lifestyle changes are total cholesterol, high-density lipoproteins (HDLs), triglycerides, and glucose.

Such preliminary information can provide valuable insights and may point up possible impairments that may cause you to limit or modify your exercise workouts. For example, elevated blood pressure may be limiting at first. You may need to walk more at the outset to see how you respond.

Whether you're tested on the treadmill or ergometer, you'll begin exercising at a low level of exertion; as the test progresses there is a systematic build-up of effort.

Throughout the testing process, the exercise electrocardiogram will be monitored on an oscilloscope. This TV-like instrument displays the electrical output of your heart. A physician or a nurse trained in advanced coronary life support should be present during graded exercise tests of high-risk or older people. If an individual being tested has hidden heart disease symptoms, the test will often provoke abnormal heart responses. Although the purpose of the test is to determine your level of physical fitness, it is not uncommon for some abnormal heart responses to occur during the test. In such cases, referral to a cardiologist or a family physician might be warranted.

Your blood pressure is regularly monitored throughout the graded exercise test to tell how the heart muscle is adapting to the increased

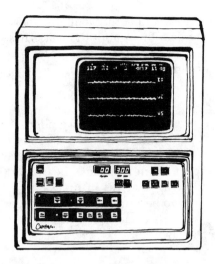

workload. A falling systolic pressure with increased workloads suggests an inability of the heart to adapt. In such cases, the testing is stopped.

The test examiners use a series of end points to stop a graded exercise test. The normal end point for apparently healthy persons is when they reach their highest levels of work tolerance. As you near the end of a graded exercise test, you reach a point at which fatigue prohibits further exertion. This stopping point is your maximal level of fitness.

The graded exercise test can be frightening at first. Going to "your max" is taxing. However, keep in mind you don't have to exercise at this level every day to get in shape. The purpose of this test is to determine your maximal capacity so your workouts can be set at a comfortable but stimulating level (usually 70 percent of your maximum capability) to ensure beneficial changes.

In some test settings, especially in research-oriented labs, the metabolic energy response to exercise is monitored and measured. During the test protocol, you are hooked up to a special valve that allows you to breathe in room air and exhale into a collection device. The content of the exhaled air is electronically measured. These measurements, along with the volume of air ventilated, are used to calculate the amount of oxygen used during each stage of the test. Eventually the maximal amount of oxygen, or energy, used is determined.

Maximal oxygen uptake can be expressed as maximal MET capacity. One MET represents the rate of energy used at rest. Therefore, maximal METs represent your highest energy capacity in multiples above rest levels. For example, a 10 MET capacity means a person has an energy capacity 10 times greater than the amount of energy used when sitting. Maximal oxygen uptake is also a measure of your functional capacity—your highest energy level reached in a graded exercise test.

Use of such sophisticated equipment also allows the constant measuring of energy cost data thoughout the test. These measures provide additional insight about one's fitness status. However, the cost of having a respiratory gas system for exercise testing may be prohibitive.

Submaximal Tests

Many testing centers use submaximal graded exercise tests to assess physical fitness. A submaximal test has a predetermined end point based on age or other parameters. Such end points are generally set at a level of 70 to 85 percent of one's maximal heart rate. A submaximal test can be useful in following changes in fitness as you progress in your exercise workouts. As you become more fit, your heart rate response to a given workload is less. The data collected can be helpful in planning individualized exercise workouts.

SELF-TESTING FOR FITNESS

Self-testing has certain advantages for persons who have no known health problems, and who have no access to (or inclination to use) testing factilties. A self-test for fitness should measure your cardiorespiratory endurance, strength, muscular endurance, and flexibility. Be accurate when taking these tests. You are only fooling yourself if you do not perform the tests properly. Record your true scores.

Some self-tests include body fat measurements, but we don't recommend you doing them yourself. If you do not take your girth measurements correctly, you could deceive yourself. Body fat can be estimated at wellness centers, fitness centers, YMCAs or YWCAs.

Cardiorespiratory Endurance Tests

To measure your cardiorespiratory endurance, you should either do a walking test—if you are over 35, overweight, and have been inactive in recent months—or a running test. Either test will enable you to select a suitable safe starting point for your cardiorespiratory endurance training.

The Walking Test

You need a stopwatch, a digital watch, or a watch with a second hand. You also need to find an area where the distance is known. Local high school tracks, YMCAs, YWCAs, and large shopping malls are good possibilities or use your car odometer to measure street distances in your neighborhood for 1, 1.5, 2, and 3 miles.

If you are going to test yourself outdoors, choose a clear day not below freezing or above 80 degrees Fahrenheit. In some areas it is necessary to walk in the early morning to avoid the heat and humidity.

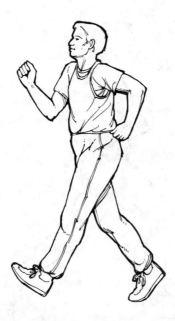

As you begin walking, start the stopwatch or note the time on your watch (it is easier if you start with the second hand on the minute mark). Walk as briskly as you can. If you begin to tire early, slow up, If you can't complete a mile, or if you can't complete it in under 25 minutes, then the test is completed.

If you walk the mile in less than 20 minutes, keep going for another half mile. If you reach the 1.5 mile point in less than 30 minutes, keep walking. Your goal is now two miles in less than 40 minutes. If you reach this goal, try to reach three miles in 60 minutes.

If you can cover the three miles in 60 minutes or less, on another day, try to run-walk a distance of two miles. This second choice may give you a more accurate idea of your capability and allow you to start at higher level on the charts.

For the run-walk test, alternate running and walking for two miles, noting the time you take to complete the distance. This test requires some heavy effort but do not exhaust yourself. After completing the two-mile run-walk, note your time. Check the fitness table to determine your estimated fitness level and starting points for the various exercise modes.

The Running Tests

The amount of time it takes you to cover a distance of 1.5 to 2 miles is an acceptable measure for approximating your maximal MET value (aerobic capacity) and fitness level. Running the distance is the best and easiest way to gain information about your fitness level if you have been

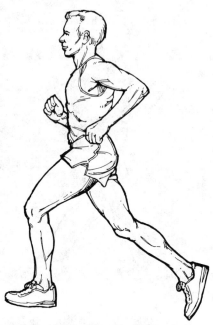

exercising regularly and haven't taken a graded exercise test. You should not engage in this test if you have been deskbound in recent years, or if you have any orthopedic problems. These tests are for people who are accustomed to running and walking the distances on a regular basis. After you have been training, you may wish to test yourself using the running test to see how you score.

For younger people and those who can run comfortably for 15 to 20 minutes continuously, being able to run 1.5 to 2 miles *all out* can provide excellent feedback on cardiorespiratory fitness. Since there are variations in aerobic capacities for men and women, two running tests are pre-

Table 3-1. 2-Mile Running Test for Men

FITNESS CATEGORY	2.0 MILE TIME	ESTIMATED MAXIMAL OXYGEN UPTAKE EQUIVALENTS	APPROXIMATE MAXIMAL METS
Super	Faster than 12:00	55 ml/kg-min or higher	15.7 Plus
Excellent	12:00 to 13:59	54.9 to 50 ml/kg-min	15.6 to 14.3
Excellent to Good	14:00 to 15:59	49.9 to 45 ml/kg-min	14.2 to 12.9
Good to Fair	16:00 to 17:59	44.9 to 40 ml/kg-min	12.8 to 11.4
Fair to Poor	18:00 to 19:59	39.9 to 35 ml/kg-min	11.3 to 10.0
Poor	20:00 or slower	34.9 or lower	9.9 or lower

Table 3-2. 1.5-Mile Running Test for Women

FITNESS CATEGORY	1.5 MILE TIME	ESTIMATED MAXIMAL OXYGEN UPTAKE EQUIVALENTS	APPROXIMATE MAXIMAL METS
Super	Faster than 11:30	52.5 ml/kg-min or higher	15 Plus
Excellent	11:30 to 12:59	52.4 to 47.5 ml/kg-min	14.9 to 13.6
Excellent to Good	13:00 to 14:29	46.4 to 42.5 ml/kg-min	13.5 to 12.1
Good to Fair	14:30 to 15:59	42.4 to 37.5 ml/kg-min	12.0 to 10.7
Fair to Poor	16:00 to 17:59	37.4 to 32.5 ml/kg-min	10.6 to 9.3
Poor	18:00 or slower	31.4 or lower	9.2 or lower

sented here. The 1.5-mile test is for women and the 2-mile test is for men.

For men, running two miles in 10 to 12 minutes is a super rating, 12 to 14 minutes is excellent, and 14 to 16 is good. For women, running 1.5 miles faster than 11.5 minutes is super, 11.5 to 13 minutes is excellent, and 13 to 14.5 minutes is good.

The times to run the 1.5-mile distance all-out for women and the two-mile distance for men correlate well with actual values of maximal oxygen uptake determined on the treadmill. Estimates of your aerobic capacity in accordance with your running times are presented in Tables 3-1 and 3-2. The data are based on young adults; however, they tend to hold true for older people as well.

Measuring Your Muscular Strength and Endurance

You can also assess your muscular strength and endurance to establish bases for improvement or to maintain your present level of fitness. This self-testing evaluates overall body strength and endurance capabilities. Caution: if you have a heart problem, do not take this test without a physician's permission.

Chapter 11 includes suggestions for developing and maintaining strength and muscular endurance.

The Sit-Up Test

The sit-up test (Figure 3-1) has been used extensively to determine the strength and endurance of the abdominal muscles. Proper technique must be followed. Research shows that holding the feet or placing them under a firm support tends to bring into play the large hip flexors of the pelvic region rather than the abdominal muscles.

Instead, lie on your back, knees bent at approximately 90 degrees, feet flat on the floor, and hands along your sides on the floor. A full sit-

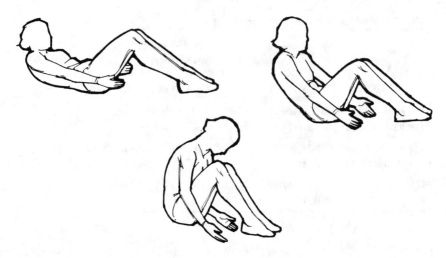

Figure 3-1. The sit-up test.

up is counted when you have curled your back and raised your trunk until your lower back is at least perpendicular to the floor and then returned to the starting position.

You will need a stopwatch, a digital watch, or a watch with a second hand. The total number of sit-ups performed in 60 seconds is your score for this test. Don't be discouraged if it is a struggle to do just one. This is common in people who have not been exercising these muscles regularly.

The Push-Up Test

The push-up (Figure 3-2) is also used extensively for measuring upper body strength and endurance. Start in a front-leaning rest position, supporting your body on your hands and toes. Lower your body by bending at the elbows until your chest touches the floor. Keep your body flat and rigid. Return to the starting position. Your score is the number of

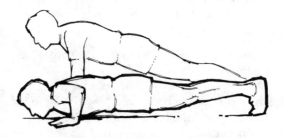

Figure 3-2. The push-up test.

Table 3-3. Muscular Strength and Endurance Standards Adult Men and Women

	SIT-UPS (60 seconds)	PUSH-UPS (60 seconds)
Excellent	30 or more	15 or more
Good	25 to 29	10 to 14
Fair	20 to 24	5 to 9
Poor	Less than 20	Less than 4

correct complete push-ups you can do in one minute. Do not despair if you cannot do even one.

Table 3-3 presents muscular endurance standards for both men and women. By including a few special exercises in each workout, you will gradually improve your strength and muscular endurance.

Measuring Your Flexibility

Flexibility is the ability to use your muscles throughout their maximum ranges of motion. Any loss of flexibility from muscle disuse limits your ability to walk smoothly, sit down or stand up gracefully, and perform your daily tasks efficiently. Chapter 5 is devoted to exercises for stretching your major muscle groups.

Although no single test result provides all the information about your flexibility level, the trunk flexion is a reasonable measure of your ability to stretch the lower back muscles and back thigh muscles (hamstrings).

Trunk Flexion Test

Sit with your legs fully extended with the bottom of your feet flat against a box projecting from the wall (Figure 3-3). The box should be at the same height as your feet. Bend your trunk while stretching your arms and hands forward as far as possible. Hold for a count of three.

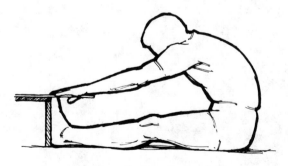

Figure 3-3. Trunk flexion test.

Table 3-4. Standards For Sit and Reach Test

	Women	Men
Normal Range	−4 to +10 in	−6 to +8 in
Average Values	+ 2 in	+1 in
Desired Range	+2 to + 6 in	+1 to +5 in

Have a partner measure in inches the distance before or beyond the edge of the box that you reach. Distances before the edge are expressed as negative scores; those beyond the edge as positive scores. Table 3-4 gives standards for flexibility.

Although this information is not used directly for planning exercise workouts, such information can provide insight into your overall fitness. It can also alert you to any impairments that could limit your exercise training.

SUMMARY

Whether you've undergone a graded exercise test or taken a self-test, you have a fairly good idea of how you "measure up". Now you can establish a personal exercise program. If you are still in doubt about your state of physical fitness, begin your program at the lowest level. You can always adjust upward.

As you progress toward fitness, retest yourself from time to time. A personal fitness profile record is provided in Table 3-5. Track your progress. Be sure to set reasonable goals. Although testing should not dominate your exercise program, it can be a worthwhile motivator for greater efforts and regular exercise habits.

Table 3-5. Personal Fitness Profile Record

	NOW Date:	3 MONTHS Date:	6 MONTHS Date:	1 YEAR Date:	2 YEARS Date:	3 YEARS Date:
Sitting Heart Rate (bts/min)						
Blood Pressure (mm/Hg)						
Body Weight						
% Body Fat						
Maximal Oxygen Uptake						
Maximal MET Level						
Distance Run (time to run 1.5 to 2 miles)						
Sit-Ups (no./min)						
Push-Ups (no.)						
Sit and Reach (in.)						

4

Basic Guidelines For Planning A Fitness Program

Many people are confused about the type and amount of exercise needed to become and stay fit. Some people who work out regularly started out improperly and found it a struggle. Fortunately, they survived the early rigors to become regular adherents. But for all those who made it, there are many more who failed. Meanwhile, fitness professionals keep hearing the same questions, which this chapter helps you answer.

- How hard do I have to exercise?
- How far do I have to run?
- Do I have to run to be physically fit?
- How long do I need to work out?
- How often do I need to work out?
- What are the best activities for getting in shape?

THE FOUR FUNDAMENTAL FACTORS

Although your fitness program should be tailored to your needs, the basic principles for achieving physical fitness are the same for all people. There are four essential ingredients for the development of a sound exercise program: 1) *intensity* (level of exertion); 2) *duration* (length of exertion); 3) *frequency* (how often); and 4) *mode* (type of activity).

Intensity: How Hard?

To improve cardiorespiratory and muscular fitness, you need to participate in a moderately intensive, physical conditioning program. This means a stimulation of the heart, lungs, and muscles, with substantial effort well within your capabilities. Remember, during exercise, the heart rate increases proportionately with the increase in energy requirements. For this reason, the exercise heart rate is used as a simple measure for estimating physiological stress on the body and is a standard means for determining exercise intensity levels.

To make appreciable gains in cardiorespiratory fitness, the heart rate during exercise (training heart rate) must be raised to near 70 percent of the difference between the resting and maximal heart rates. This is referred to as your 70 percent heart rate (HR) reserve. Exercising somewhere between 60 and 80 percent heart rate reserve represents a safe and reasonable intensity for most people.

How to Count Your Pulse

To determine your training or target heart rate, you must know your heart rate at rest. And, to determine your exercise intensity, you need to know your heart rate immediately after exercise. Except in rare cases, the number of heartbeats each minute is equal to the number of pulse beats each minute. Therefore, your heart rate can be counted at any convenient pulse point.

Follow these steps to determine your pulse rate. Get a stopwatch or a wristwatch with a second hand. Locate your most suitable pulse point. By placing the tips of the fingers on your chest, below and to the side of your left nipple, you can generally pick up your heartbeat. Or try your carotid artery, which is located just under your jaw bone on your neck slightly behind your Adam's apple. Taking your pulse on the inside of your wrist may be the best site. Place the tips of two fingers immediately below the base of the thumb. Be sure to press lightly (Figure 4-1). When you feel your pulse, count the beats for 30 seconds. Then multiply your 30-second pulse rate by two to determine your pulse in beats per minute.

It is easy to determine your heart rate at rest: just sit down and take your pulse. It is, however, a little more difficult to take your pulse during exercise. For practical purposes assume the rate counted immediately following exercise is equivalent to the exercising rate. Immediately after exercise, the pulse rate declines rapidly, so it is important for you to learn to count your pulse within a second or two after stopping. The pulse beats will be rapid and strong, thus easier to locate. Count your pulse for 10 seconds, then multiply by six.

It may take a little practice before you can consistently obtain a reliable pulse rate. Through experimenting, you can find your most reliable pulse point.

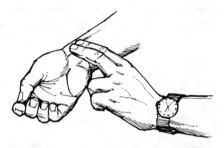

Figure 4-1. Pulse counting at wrist.

Determining Your Target Heart Rate

Determining your target or training heart rate is simple. Take the difference between your maximal and sitting rates, multiply it by .70 (70 percent HR reserve). Add the result to your sitting rate.

The maximal heart rate for most adults generally ranges between 160 and 200 beats per minute. This value represents your highest attainable heart rate. (See Chapter 2.) It has little relationship to your state of fitness. Although it is best determined by a graded exercise test (see Chapter 3), it can be estimated to be 220 minus your age. To estimate your training heart rate, use the formula below.

For example, use a maximal heart rate of 180 (an estimate for a 40-year-old) and a sitting rate of 80. The difference is 100 beats. Seventy percent of 100 is 70 beats. Adding this figure to the resting rate of 80, we get a target heart rate of 150 beats (approximately 25 beats for 10 seconds). This figure represents 70 percent HR reserve, a safe and effective training level for that person. Similar calculations for a maximal heart rate of 200 (a value for a young adult) would result in a target heart rate of 170.

When engaging in physical activity, you need to exercise close to your training heart rate to produce significant cardiorespiratory benefits. Don't worry about how fast you walk, swim, or run. Just try to stay near your target heart rate. For most adults, this intensity means a target heart rate in the range of 140 to 170 beats per minute.

For older adults, because of a decline in maximal heart rate with aging, a lower heart rate may represent an adequate training stimulus. A rate of 120 to 140 beats per minute may suffice. When you exercise at approximately a 70 percent effort, you should be able to keep a conversation going. If you can't talk, you are probably working out too intensely. For some people, it may be wise to exercise at a 50 to 60 percent heart rate reserve. This is true for people with an excessive weight problem.

Table 4-1 presents a chart for converting 10-second pulse counts to beats per minute. For example, 26 beats for 10 seconds is equivalent to an exercise heart rate of 156.

Duration: How Long?

The duration of exercise is directly related to the intensity of the activity. Exertion at your target heart rate enables you to spread your workout session over a longer period of time than is allowed by a more intense level of exercise.

The Three-Segment Workout

Most workouts for developing physical fitness consist of three essential parts: 1) the warm-up; 2) the main vigorous conditioning period;

Table 4-1. Conversion of 10-Second Pulse Counts to Heart Rate

10-Second Pulse Counts	Heart Rate Beats/Minute
15	90
16	96
17	102
18	108
19	114
20	120
21	126
22	132
23	138
24	144
25	150
26	156
27	162
28	168
29	174
30	180

and 3) the cool-down. All three segments are necessary for a sound program. (Figure 4-2).

Another essential component to an overall fitness program is strength and muscular endurance exercises. While aerobic- type exercises condition the cardiorespiratory system, strength and muscular endurance exercises condition another key component of the body—the muscles. See Chapter 11.

The Warm-Up

Proper warm-up before each workout is wise. In addition to preparing your body for exertion, the warm-up is a precaution against unnecessary injuries and muscle soreness. It progressively stimulates

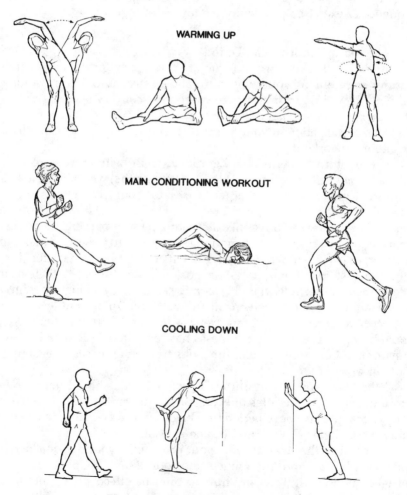

Figure 4-2. Three-segment workout.

the heart and lungs, increases the blood flow, and gradually increases the temperatures of the blood and muscles. A complete warm-up stretches the muscles and tendons in preparation for more forceful contractions. It also prepares you mentally for strenuous activities. You should experience an overall feeling of well-being as you complete your preparation.

How long should you warm-up? The time varies with the individual. As soon as you begin to sweat (an indication that the temperature of the deep tissues has increased), you are probably ready for the more intense conditioning workout. If you are outside, cool weather requires longer warm-up times.

Because of the importance of the warm-up, a complete chapter has been devoted to proper warm up and stretching. Chapter 5 presents a sequence of exercises you could use for warming up.

The Main Conditioning Period

After a sufficient warm-up, you are now ready for the main conditioning segment of your workout. The best activities are walking, running, bicycling, swimming, rowing, cross-country skiing, aerobics, and other rhythmical, large muscle activities. As you get in better shape, vigorous participation in your favorite sport can be used occasionally as an alternate workout.

If you alternate periods of vigorous exercise with exercise of lower intensity (*you will learn how to do this in later chapters*), you will be able to keep from going over your target heart rate. Your peak efforts should never exceed 85 to 90 percent HR reserve. However, when you reach the point where your workout omits alternating periods of exercise and rest, as in continuous running or swimming, it is easier to judge and maintain your target heart rate without much fluctuation. It is common for those who can sustain running for 30 or more minutes to elevate their heart rate to the 80 percent level and be comfortable. In a walking program, it is unlikely you can elevate your heart rate to the 70 percent level.

Most research suggests an exercise session of 30 minutes is long enough to produce beneficial fitness changes. There is some additional enhancement in cardiovascular functions from training sessions of up to an hour or more.

When you embark on a fitness program, you should not exercise continuously for 30 minutes or even reach a 70 percent level. Limit your early workouts to short periods of vigorous exercise alternated with more moderate levels of exercise such as walking.

Remember, the key is to tailor your program to your personal needs. Most people want to do too much, too soon. Many people believe the mistaken notion, "if it doesn't hurt, it can't be effective." Do not force yourself to suffer. Our approach to exercise training is to stay well within your capabilities at an intensity sufficient for improvement and maintenance.

As your fitness improves over time, it will be possible to modify your workout and increase the total work accomplished in each session.

The workout should always be set so you feel fully recovered and rested within an hour after its completion. At the start, your workout may last only 20 minutes, but gradually you will become accustomed to longer periods of vigorous exercise at the proper intensity level.

The Cool-Down

The cool-down is a tapering off period after your main workout. It is best accomplished by continued activity at a lower intensity. Some highly trained individuals use intermittent running at a lower tempo as a cooling-down procedure. However, walking is a more common practice. You can also repeat some of the warm-up exercises during the cool-down.

Tapering off allows your muscles to assist in pumping the blood from the extremities back to the heart. If you end a workout abruptly, your heart continues to send extra blood to the muscles for a few minutes. Since the muscles are no longer contracting and helping to propel the blood back to the central circulation, blood may pool in the muscles. As a result, there may be insufficient blood for the other organs. In fact, if you don't keep moving you may experience dizziness.

Keep moving to help your breathing and heart rate return to near normal before you head for a shower. Generally, a five-to-10 minute recovery period is sufficient under normal conditions. For most participants, the heart rate at the end of the cool-down should be below 100.

Frequency: How Often?

Regular adherence to a vigorous exercise program is necessary if you are to reach and maintain an adequate level of physical fitness. Training effects are gained and lost rather quickly.

Daily physical activity, though desirable, is not necessary to improve or maintain cardiorespiratory fitness. *Above-average cardiorespiratory fitness can be attained with regular workouts four times per week.* Keep in mind, however, that improvements in many aspects of physical fitness occur over many months. It is wise to allow several of the initial weeks for adaptation. This recommendation is based on the assumption that your workouts will eventually be at your target heart rate intensity for at least 30 minutes.

Mode of Activity: What Kind?

The relative values of various activities for improving physical fitness depend on the physiological intensity required. Activities *low in intensity and short in duration* produce low levels of improvement. For instance, golf, bowling, and softball do little to develop or maintain physical fitness. While these activities are great fun, they do not provide the necessary physiological stimulus for fitness.

Moderately intensive, continuous, and rhythmic activities involving the large muscle groups (brisk walking, running, cycling, and swimming) are excellent for the development of the entire body. Such activities force the heart to beat at a rhythmic rate high enough to challenge your cardiorespiratory system. Incorporating strength and muscular endurance exercises like sit-ups and push-ups into your weekly workouts will ensure overall physical fitness.

In general, activities requiring short bursts of speed and quick movements do little to improve your cardiorespiratory system. For example, playing racquetball or tennis, even 30 to 60 minutes four days a week, is not as beneficial as rhythmic, activities for substantial physical fitness. Obviously, the skill of the participant determines the training benefit of any sports activity. If you and your opponent are competent players, you may be able to stay active enough to keep your heart rate elevated for conditioning purposes. However, a sustained workout for 30 minutes at a 60 to 80 percent HR reserve intensity four days a week will produce greater cardiorespiratory fitness. Such workouts will better prepare you for a racquetball or tennis game. You don't get in shape by playing a sport; you get in shape to play your favorite sport.

If you have been inactive, avoid these highly competitive sports. The older you get, the more dangerous quick movements and sudden bursts of energy become unless you have been participating regularly in appropriate physical fitness activities.

VARYING INTENSITY, DURATION, FREQUENCY, AND MODE

There is a direct relationship between the degree of cardiorespiratory improvement and the intensity, duration, and frequency of the workout sessions. These factors can be varied to reach the same results.

Age, medical limitations, excess body weight, or a combination of these may make it necessary to vary the intensity and duration components. If you can't work out at your training heart rate, then you will need more frequent workouts five to six times a week at a lower intensity and for a longer duration (45 to 60 minutes).

Older individuals and excessively overweight people begin with walking as their main exercise mode. Even with brisk walking, it is difficult to elevate your heart rate intensity unless you are able to walk up a steep incline on a treadmill. Thus, walking requires a longer exercise period to achieve fitness gains.

For people starting out, we strongly recommend a four-day-a-week exercise schedule to lessen the chance of injury during the early stages of training. After your body adapts to regular bouts of exercise you may want to add a fifth day. Or, you may want to alternate aerobic activities with strength and endurance development. By varying your exercise routine, you will reduce the chances of injury, increase motivation, and develop the strength and endurance of the muscle groups.

Remember, your goal is to achieve the results obtained by reaching a target heart rate of 70 percent of your heart rate reserve, for 30 minutes, four days a week, in addition to good warm-up and cool down periods. Working out at a lower heart rate requires an upward adjustment in duration, frequency, or both. Likewise, shorter exercise periods must be balanced with more workouts.

When choosing a mode, you must know how hard, how long, and how often to work out to get the desired results. The information provided in Chapters 6 through 9 will help you choose from a variety of modes. Once you have learned how you respond to various modes, you can better adjust your intensity, duration, and frequency.

SUMMARY

Working between 60 to 80 percent of your HR reserve is mostly aerobic, so do not worry about how fast you go. Your heart's response to your workout should be your main concern. Whether you want to walk, run, cycle, or swim, the programs and charts outlined in this book are designed for you. You must be willing to devote the necessary time and effort to your fitness training if you want to reap the benefits.

Today, nearly everyone preaches the virtues of physical fitness, yet many do not maintain a regular fitness program. Two primary reasons for this failure are not knowing: 1) how much exercise is enough, and 2) the kinds of exercise that work best for physical fitness.

Many writers on physical fitness have neglected to take firm stands on recommending physical fitness activities. One frequently hears such vague statements as, "There are many ways to develop fitness," "Do your own thing," "Choose whatever activity you enjoy," or "Don't sweat." Such suggestions are groundless and confusing. Of course there are different ways to develop cardiorespiratory fitness. Nevertheless, you must exert yourself, *in a continuous and rhythmic activity at a substantial level of exertion for at least 30 minutes*. And you must adhere to this program regularly.

Let's be clear about it: it takes effort to be physically fit. This does not mean punishing, exhaustive exercise, but rather a workout that is well within your present physical capacity.

The exercise charts have been developed from our knowledge and experience of what it takes for individuals to become fit, regardless of their present physical states. These charts represent carefully planned steps to guide you through the early stages of getting in shape, and most importantly, at an intensity that is right for you. Eventually you will reach the point where you will not need the charts. You will be ready to assume the responsibility of continuing your own workouts and maintaining your new status of being fit.

5

The Importance of Stretching and Muscle Toning

Toning and stretching exercises should be an integral part of a well-rounded physical fitness program. The warm-up segment of a workout is the best time to stretch the major muscle groups and to do some muscle-toning exercises. In his book, *Stretching*, Bob Anderson writes "stretching feels good when done correctly, and it reduces muscular tension and promotes freer movement."

Stretching is not stressful. It is peaceful, relaxing, and non-competitive. You do not have to conform to any unyielding discipline; stretching gives you the freedom to enjoy yourself.

Stretching and muscle-toning exercises are important before workouts for two reasons: they help stretch and tone the muscles, and they gradually prepare the cardiorespiratory system.

Many people believe muscle-toning exercises will trim unwanted inches off their waists or hips. Unfortunately, despite what many so-called experts claim, there is no concrete evidence that exercising a particular spot of the body will take off inches. Inches slowly come off at the fatty sites only when the body's metabolic rate is increased substantially on a regular basis.

Many people believe physical fitness is reflected only in external appearance. They have the mistaken notion that if you look fit, you are fit. A trim and firm body, a radiant complexion, and youthful vigor come not only from exercise that improves muscle tone, but also from activities that stress the cardiorespiratory system. Physical fitness, with the extra benefits of fat loss and improved body proportions, requires a vigorous stimulation of the heart, lungs, and muscles. Stretching and toning exercises are just one part of a total conditioning program.

THE WARM-UP

The following Fitness 12 exercises can easily be incorporated into your fitness program. The exercises serve as a means of loosening, stretching, shaping, and strengthening your major muscle groups.

You may have your own set of warm-ups similar to the ones presented here. There's no reason to stop doing them. Just be sure they are stretching and toning most of your major muscle groups. You might try these to see how you like them.

The sequence of warm-ups is a combination of conventional and some of the newer yoga-type, calisthenic exercises. Yoga involves holding a static position for a period of time. Such a posture puts the stretched muscles and connective tissues at the desired length without causing injury. Static stretching, as this method is often called, is very effective. Bouncy movements impose strain on the involved muscles and cause reflexes that actually oppose the desired stretching. So stretch slowly. Be careful to stretch the muscles to a point of tension where it feels good, and you feel a slight pull. Overstretching, especially if done with rapid movements, can lead to injury.

Many of the leg-stretching exercises should be repeated during the cool-down phase of your workout. Brisk walking, cycling, and especially running do little to develop flexibility. In fact, daily running can even harm your leg muscles. Runners often experience abnormal tightening of the hamstrings (the back muscles of the thigh). This can lead to strength imbalances. Running requires a relatively small range of movements. When the leg muscles are used repeatedly over a sustained period, they tend to become very tight. By stretching your muscles before and after each workout you decrease your chances of injuries.

Although these exercises were primarily developed for stretching before and after a conditioning workout, try to stretch whenever you get the opportunity. Stretching is a form of relaxation—it can help you avoid tight muscles any time, and it may even refresh you.

The muscle-toning exercises, such as arm-swinging, are designed to promote full range of motion as well as some muscle development. Be sure to do these rhythmically and at a moderate tempo.

Before doing the warm-ups, a few minutes of walking are recommended. This is especially important before beginning an early morning workout. This will get your heart pumping and blood flowing. After you've been up and around, the need for preliminary walking is not as important.

The Instructions for the Fitness 12

Do these stretching exercises at your own tempo. They are presented in a progressive, easy-to-follow sequence. The purpose of each exercise is explained. Besides illustrating the movements, starting positions are presented. Three levels of exertion—light, moderate, and heavy—are suggested for each activity. The appropriate number of repetitions are indicated. Begin with the lightest level and work toward the moderate and heavy.

Remember: avoid bobbing or forcing your body into unaccustomed positions. If you haven't been exercising regularly, it will take time before you can stretch some of those tight muscles completely. Don't hurry. If you proceed at a comfortable pace, you will gradually accomplish what you want—more flexibility and better muscle tone. The key is to warm up your body and muscles for the upcoming workout.

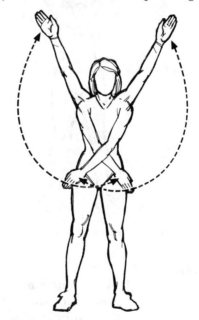

Figure 5-1. Arm circles—inward cross.

1. **Arm Circles**

   Purpose: To loosen and stretch the muscles of the arms and shoulder region.

   Starting Position: Stand with your feet shoulder-width apart and your arms at your sides.

   Movement: In each of the four following exercises, your arms should make large, sweeping circles. Keep your elbows straight and swing your arms from the shoulders.

Inward Cross-body: Swing your arms inward, upward, and around crossing in front of the face and body (Figure 5-1).

10	15	20
Light	Moderate	Heavy

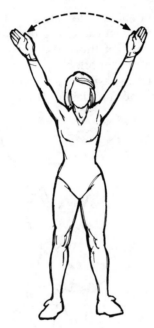

Figure 5-2. Arm circles—outward cross.

Outward Cross Body:

Swing your arms outward, upward, and around, crossing in front of your body and above your head (Figure 5-2).

10	15	20
Light	Moderate	Heavy

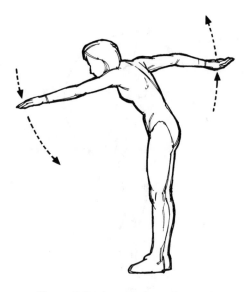

Figure 5-3. Arm circles—forward.

Forward: Swing your arms forward, as in a crawl
                      swimming motion. Make large sweeping
                      circles alternately. Count a complete circle
                      with the left and right arm as one revolu-
                      tion (Figure 5-3).

10	15	20
Light	Moderate	Heavy

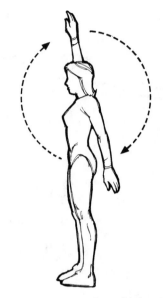

Figure 5-4. Arm circles—backward.

Backward: Swing your arms backward alternately as
                          in a backward swimming crawl. Make
                          large sweeping circles (Figure 5-4).

10	15	20
Light	Moderate	Heavy

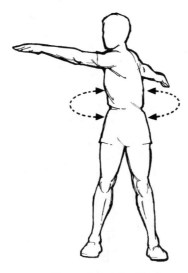

Figure 5-5. Trunk twister.

2. **Trunk Twister**

Purpose: To loosen and stretch muscles in the back,
                       side, and shoulder region.

Starting Position: Start with your feet shoulder-width apart,
                       arms extended to the sides at shoulder
                       level.

Movement: While keeping your heels flat on the floor
                       with toes straight ahead, twist your trunk
                       to the right slowly as far as you can turn.
                       Then return to the starting position. Now
                       twist slowly to the left. Repeat the com-
                       plete movement slowly (Figure 5-5).

6	9	12
Light	Moderate	Heavy

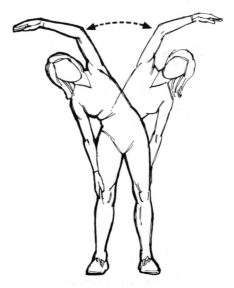

Figure 5-6. Shoulder and groin stretch.

3. Side and Groin Stretcher

Purpose:	To loosen and stretch the side muscles of the trunk and groin area.
Starting Position:	With your feet shoulder-width apart, extend one arm upward (palm facing inward) and the other arm downward (palm touching the side of your thigh).
Movement:	Bend your truck to the side of the lower extended arm. Reach with your lower hand and stretch, sliding the hand down your thigh to the knee or lower. The other arm should be stretched over your head and in the direction of body's lean. Return to the starting position and repeat the exercise on the other side (Figure 5-6). Alternate.

3	5	6
Light	Moderate	Heavy

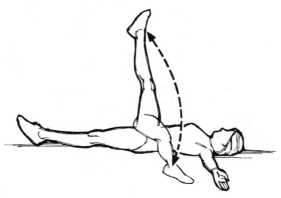

Figure 5-7. Leg-over.

4. **Leg-Overs**

Purpose: To loosen and stretch the rotator muscles of the lower back and the pelvic region.

Starting Position: Lie on your back with your legs extended, and your arms extended at shoulder level (palms up).

Movement: Keep the knee extended as you raise one leg to a vertical position (point your toes). The opposite leg should remain on the floor in extended position; keep the back of that leg on the floor. While keeping your shoulders, arms, and back on the floor, reach with the vertically extended leg across your body to the extended opposite hand. Stretch to touch your toe to the floor in the area of the extended hand. Then return your leg first to the vertical position and then to the floor (Figure 5-7). Follow the same procedure with the other leg. Repeat the complete exercise.

4	6	8
Light	Moderate	Heavy

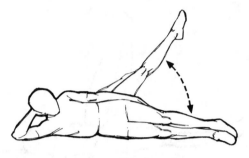

Figure 5-8. Side-leg raises.

5. Side Leg Raises

Purpose:	To strengthen and stretch the lateral hip muscles.
Starting Position:	Lie on your right side, in extended position, with your head resting on your right forearm and hand.
Movement:	Raise your left leg upward from the floor (keeping the knee extended and toes drawn up toward the center of your body) to a position well above the horizontal. Return to the starting position. Keep your pelvis perpendicular to the floor (Figure 5-8). After completing the repetitions for one side, repeat the exercise on the other side.

10	15	20
Light	Moderate	Heavy

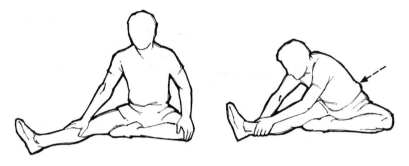

Figure 5-9. Hamstring stretch.

6. Hamstring Stretch

Purpose:	To stretch the hamstrings.
Starting Position:	While sitting down, straighten the right leg with the sole of your left foot slightly touching the inside of the right thigh.
Movement:	Slowly bend forward from the hips toward the foot of the straight leg until you create the slightest feeling of stretch in the rear thigh muscles (Figure 5-9). Continue to breathe normally and hold for 20 to 30 seconds. Then switch sides.
Caution:	Keep the foot of the straight leg upright with the ankle and toes relaxed. Be sure the quadriceps are relaxed during the stretch. Bend from the hips rather than dipping your head forward when initiating the stretch.

(per side)

2	4	6
Light	Moderate	Heavy

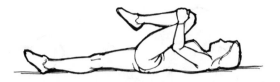

Figure 5-10. Low back stretcher.

7. Low-Back Stretcher

Purpose:	To stretch and loosen the lower back and hip flexor muscles.
Starting Position:	Lie on your back with your knees straight.
Movement:	Pull one knee to your chest. Grasp the leg just below the knee and pull the knee toward your chest (Figure 5-10). Continue to breathe normally and hold for 10 or more seconds. Return to starting position and repeat the exercise with the other leg. Alternate.

4	6	8
Light	Moderate	Heavy

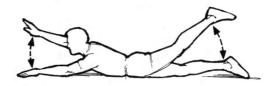

Figure 5-11. Arm and leg lifter.

8. Arm and Leg Lifter

Purpose:	To strengthen and stretch the extensor muscles of the back and hip.
Starting Position:	Lie face down (prone position) with your arms extended over your head and your legs extended.
Movement:	Raise your right arm and left leg, toes pointed, simultaneously and keep them extended for a few seconds. Then return to the starting position. Now raise the left arm and right leg simultaneously (Figure 5-11). Alternate. Do this exercise slowly. Be sure not to overextend. Do not jerk your legs and arms.

4	6	8
Light	Moderate	Heavy

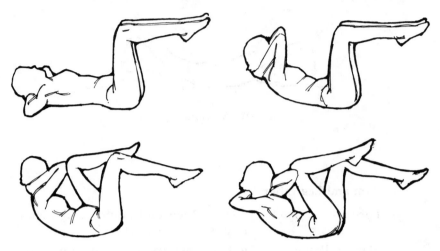

Figure 5-12. Abdominal curl.

9. **Abdominal Curl**

Purpose:	To strengthen and tone the abdominal muscles.
Starting Position:	Lie on your back with knees bent and feet flat on the floor. Put your hands behind your head, elbows pointing ahead. Raise the bent knees toward the chest so thighs are perpendicular to the floor.
Movement:	As you curl up, bring the right elbow toward the left knee. Then bring the left knee back toward it (Figure 5-12). Then left elbow to right knee. Repeat this six times to each knee. Do three sets. (When performing this exercise avoid pulling on the neck, which tends to put pressure on the cervical spine.)

6	8	10
Light	Moderate	Heavy

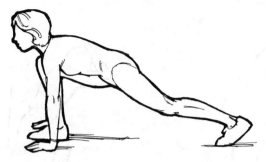

Figure 5-13. Stride stretcher.

10. Stride Stretcher

Forward position

Purpose:	To stretch the lower back muscles, hip flexors, and leg muscles.
Starting Position:	Move one leg forward so it is flexed under your chest. The knee should be directly over the ankle, and your other leg should be stretched out behind. Your arms and bent leg must be in line with each other, perpendicular to the floor.
Movement:	With both hands on the floor and your forward heel on the floor, roll your body forward while pushing your hips down toward the floor (Figure 5-13). Continue to breathe normally and hold for 10 or more seconds. Repeat the exercise with the other leg forward.

5	10	15
Light	Moderate	Heavy

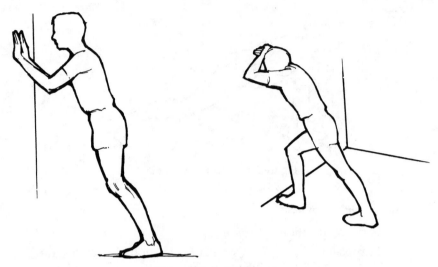

Figure 5-14. Calf stretcher.

11. Calf Stretcher, Leaning

Purpose:	To stretch your calf muscles.
Starting Position:	Stand 20 inches from a solid support. Lean on it with your forearms, head resting on hands.
Movement:	Bend one leg and place your foot on the ground in front of you. Keep the other leg straight behind you. Slowly move your hips forward, keeping your lower back flat. Be sure to keep the heel of the straight leg on the ground, with toes pointed straight ahead or slightly turned in as you hold the stretch (Figure 5-14). Hold an easy stretch for 20 to 30 seconds. Stretch the other leg.

2	4	6
Light	Moderate	Heavy

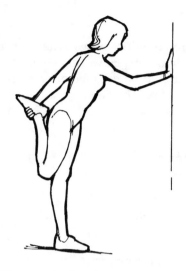

Figure 5-15. Standing quad stretcher.

12. Standing Quad Stretcher

Purpose:	To stretch the quadriceps. Also expands chest and stretches shoulder muscles.
Starting Position:	While standing erect and keeping your back straight, bend the right knee and lift the right foot directly behind the body. Hold the toes of the foot with the left hand. Use your right hand to balance on a wall or chair.
Movement:	Bend the lifted right knee and draw the leg up and back. Pull up the right leg until you feel a slight discomfort in the upper front thigh (quadricep muscles) (Figure 5-15). Balance and hold firmly for five or more seconds. (It is important to keep your back straight while holding the stretch). Repeat with the other leg.

2	4	6
Light	Moderate	Heavy

THE QUICK SIX

The Fitness 12 are sound exercises. They can be done easily and safely. You can even add others. However, when you are in a hurry, here are six exercises that should be done before a workout to avoid injury. We call them the Quick Six. They are:

1. Arm swings
2. Trunk twister
3. Lower back stretch
4. Hamstring stretcher
5. Achilles and calf stretcher
6. Standing quad stretcher

SUMMARY DO'S AND DON'TS

1. Do warm up by doing stretching and toning exercises before a workout. Stretching helps to avoid injuries.
2. Do each exercise slowly and smoothly without jerking. This prevents injuries due to overstretching.
3. Do hold each stretching position for 10 to 30 seconds, remembering to breathe normally.
4. Don't strain. Go to the edge of your stretch until you feel a slight to moderate pull. If the stretch causes pain or increasing discomfort, back off until it does not hurt.
5. Do stretch after your workout and other times during the day. This helps keep your major muscle groups from tightening up.

Part II

Moderately Intense Exercise

The following five chapters offer specific exercise prescriptions to help you plan an individualized program for developing and maintaining cardiorespiratory endurance. The paramount emphasis of the programs is to condition the heart, lungs, and blood vessels and to improve the ability to deliver oxygen to the muscle tissues. Rhythmic, moderately intense exercises sustained for a minimum of 30 minutes are the best activities for improving the cardiorespiratory functions.

A word of caution. Although exercise is beneficial, it can lead to injuries. Common sense can help you avoid problems. Many injuries are the result of overuse—doing too much, too soon. This is why you should follow the recommendations and charts in each specific activity. It is common for enthusiastic devotees to ignore these suggestions and begin increasing the length of the workouts on their own. An extra lap or two can lead to injury.

Don't forget to stretch before and after each workout. As you increase your capabilities, you will find it necessary to stretch more during the warm-up and cool-down. The Fitness 12 or similar stretching and toning exercises need to be a regular part of every workout.

6

Walking

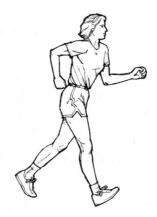

Walking is a natural and healthy form of exercise.

For many people who want to exercise, walking should be their first (and for many, their main) activity. This is especially true for older people and individuals who have been inactive. Regardless of your age, if you are extremely overweight, walking is your wisest choice.

Many authorities say walking is the best form of exercise. Walking does not place a heavy strain on the tendons of the foot and leg, and it helps beginners avoid injury in the early stages of training.

Once your body adjusts to sustained brisk walking on a regular basis, and you lose some weight (if you need to), you may want to include some running in your workout. If you are unable to run due to special medical limitations, walking represents an effective way to develop and maintain a lifelong fitness program.

WHAT WALKING CAN AND CAN'T DO FOR YOU

Fitness walking is done at a brisk walking pace with a full swing of the arms at a rate that stimulates the heart and lungs. At first you may not be able to maintain this pace. Eventually, you should cover a mile every 15 minutes or less for 45 minutes to an hour.

If you want to reap significant fitness changes on a walking program, you must walk for longer than the 30 minutes recommended for running, cycling, and swimming. Walking is lower in intensity, so as you get in better shape, you cannot walk fast enough to reach your target heart rate. If, however, you are able to do your walking on a treadmill, you can increase the intensity by increasing the incline. Walking up an incline while maintaining a brisk pace is the only way you can get benefits similar to those gained through running.

WHERE TO WALK

Try to choose a place with a stable and smooth surface. Walk where it is safe; if you walk at night or in the early morning, always carry a flashlight. Avoid automobile traffic.

Many people have discovered "mall walking." It is easy and safe, and it offers companionship, interesting sights, and controlled temperatures. Many malls have encouraged walkers and have even offered special programs sponsored by the American Heart Association. Remember to walk briskly to stimulate the blood flow. Window shop while you cool down!

Walking is usually an outdoor activity, and in most cases, it is not difficult to determine how far you walk. You can easily determine mileage by using a car's odometer. Some of you will probably take advantage of a track; most outdoor tracks are 440 yards (a quarter of a mile) around. However, indoor tracks are seldom longer than 220 yards (an eighth of a mile). At times, distance may have to be estimated, especially if you use a shopping mall. But keeping track of the time you walk will give you some indication.

WHAT TO WEAR

Walking requires a minimum of equipment and clothing. Your single largest investment is in footgear (Figure 6-1). Any activity in which force is applied to the feet, ankles, and knees can cause problems. The heavier you are, the greater the possibility of injury. Depending on the type of walking and the terrain, your footwear can range from jogging shoes to hiking boots.

Canvas tennis sneakers and racquetball or basketball shoes will not do. They do not give the support needed for walking briskly for an hour or more.

Jogging shoes make excellent walking shoes on easy-to- cover and relatively smooth ground. They have good multi-layered soles, strong

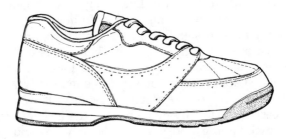

Figure 6-1. Walking footgear.

heel counters, and flexible forefoots. The built-in arch supports are helpful, especially if you have low arches.

Lightweight walking shoes, made from leather or canvas, are fine on smooth terrain and in cross-country and mountainous areas. Shoe manufacturers are now making some excellent all-round lightweight walking shoes.

When you shop for your shoes, try on more than one pair. Walk around in them. Many athletic and footgear stores will allow you to walk or jog outside so you can feel how the shoe behaves on the pavement. They should feel so good you want to get started immediately.

Whatever type of walking shoe you choose, socks are an important adjunct. Medium or heavyweight athletic socks absorb perspiration, keep your feet comfortable during walking, and absorb shock.

Wear comfortable clothing. A general rule is to wear as little as you can. In hot, humid weather, wear light-colored loose-fitting clothing that is porous enough to allow your body to breathe. Cotton, or a combination of cotton and polyester, are your best bets. Cotton absorbs sweat and allows for easy sweat evaporation. The key is not to trap heat or moisture. You want to avoid excessive dehydration, possible heat exhaustion, and heat stroke.

In contrast, in cold weather you want to trap the warm air coming off your body and hold it. Therefore, dress in layers. Keep the chest and rib cage warm with several thin layers, one shirt being a turtleneck. For example, wear a T-shirt, turtleneck, and a nylon windbreaker. The outer layer (windbreaker) should be easy to unzip and take off as your body warms. As you walk with the wind to your back, you may need to open your jacket; however, when you turn into the wind, you may need to close it. Be sure to wear mittens and a stocking cap to keep the fingers and ears protected from frostbite. A cap also prevents you from losing valuable body heat. If you are still cold, add another layer of clothing, not heavier garments.

HOW TO WALK

You need to learn how to walk for fitness. At first, walk at a comfortable, natural, and rhythmic pace. Put a rhythm in your walk and let your arms swing in a relaxed way (Figure 6-2). Stand tall with your head high. Let your heel hit first and roll on to the ball of your foot. Keep your walking motion a relaxed glide, with your legs swinging forward freely from your hip sockets, eliminating the rolling motions of the buttocks as your leg advances.

After a few sessions, your muscles and breathing will begin to adjust to your walking pace. Increase your distance a little every day. Eventually, as you get in better shape, you can pick up the tempo.

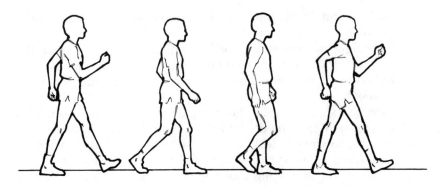

Figure 6-2. Walking motions.

Lengthen your stride and arm swing. The idea is not to be breathless but to be breathing faster and with greater depth than you do at rest. Your pace should be brisk and always challenging to your cardiorespiratory system. Be aware of how close you are to your target heart rate. If you find it difficult to maintain the your pace, slow down for about a minute to recover before returning to your training pace. Alternating brisk walking with slower walking can allow you to sustain your workout and to accomplish your distance goal for the day.

REGULATING YOUR WALKING INTENSITY

After you have walked for as little as 10 minutes, stop and check your pulse. It is always important to check your pulse within a second or two after you stop exercising. If you don't, your count will not accurately reflect your exercise heart rate. This may be difficult at first, but with a little practice it becomes easy. (See page 48 on how to take your pulse.)

The key is to exercise near your target rate. For most people, even those with a low level of fitness, it is unlikely that a target heart rate of 70 percent of heart rate reserve can be reached as a result of walking. However, some people walking at a good pace can reach 60 percent. Combining this intensity level with lengthening the workout eventually to an hour provides a good stimulus for improving cardiorespiratory fitness.

Check your pulse rate after you have cooled down for five to 10 minutes. At this point your pulse should be near 100 or below. If not, you may have worked too hard. Lack of sleep, illness, and climatic conditions, (high humidity and temperature), can affect your heart rate not only during but after your workout.

As you progress, it may not be necessary to check your pulse every day. With experience, you will be more attuned to the sensation of exercise. You will find you can estimate your level of intensity without taking your pulse. For many, it is fun and intriguing to see how the heart responds to training. As you become better trained, you will note a lower heart rate at the end of your walk. This is a good sign you are ready to pick up your pace.

AVOID INJURIES

Most walking injuries come from *overuse*. Progress slowly and gradually. Too little is better than too much at the start of your program. It is common to experience some aches and pains as you begin, but if you stick with the suggested sequence of walking workouts, any aches will last only a few days.

If pain persists in the toes or ankles or in the joints of the knees, hips, or lower back, there could be reason for concern. Make certain you have good cushion and support in your shoes. If you have flat feet, you may need some kind of arch support. Persistent pain should be reported to your exercise leader, or you should see a specialist such as a sports podiatrist or an orthopedic doctor who is familiar with athletic injuries.

SELECTING A STARTING POINT

Our walking program is set up for most middle-aged and older people, especially those who are at low levels of fitness. It will help to know your fitness level so you can select a safe starting point for your fitness walking program. If you did not take any test, start with Chart 1, Step 1.

THE WALKING CHARTS

The walking charts have three parts. No matter where you begin on the charts, start with a warm-up of stretching exercises as described in Chapter 5.

Chart 6-1 is the starter program, which goes for 16 sessions, approximately four weeks. After completing this chart, you should move to Chart 6-2, the intermediate program, for an additional four weeks. After completing Chart 6-2, you are ready for Chart 6-3, the advanced program. The box on page 83 contains a summary of instructions for using the walking charts.

The charts are just guidelines. They have been used for years and have worked for many people. Nevertheless, at times you may need to modify a day's workout, depending on how you feel. Suppose you cannot complete the prescribed walking distance for that day. When you resume the program, repeat the previous day's workout until you can complete it.

On the other hand, some people adapt to the walking workouts more rapidly than others. As long as you proceed with caution, feel free to modify the program to suit your progress.

Keep a record of your progress through the charts. As you complete each walking session, check the appropriate box on the chart and record your peak training heart rate. You may want to note your heart rate at the end of your walking session.

Four walking workouts a week are recommended. Many people prefer a Monday-Tuesday-Thursday-Friday pattern. You do not need to exercise every day; however, many walkers walk five to six days a week. At the outset follow the four-day pattern.

Rest days are important in all stages of training. Rest days allow your body to recover and adjust to the training stimulus. After your body adjusts to the four-day workout, you may want to add another day to your weekly schedule.

If you miss one or more sessions, you will need to make some adjustments when you resume your workouts. If you missed only a day or two, you may only need to drop back one session below the last one completed. If you missed a week or more, you need to make a greater adjustment. Do not be tempted to disregard this advice. Failure to drop back may lead to unnecessary injuries and could endanger your health.

Your goal is to walk two miles comfortably. Once you have adjusted, you can strive to increase your distance, then to walk the distance faster.

Once you are able to walk a brisk three to four miles, you are ready to vary your workouts. Find a new place to walk or vary your distances. One day, for example, you might walk five miles or more; the next day you could stride out on a three-mile walk at better than a 15-minute-mile pace. Innovations such as these will help diversify your walks. Your ability to walk four or more miles in an hour or less is a respectable accomplishment. Once accomplished, you may want to consider integrating some short running bouts into your workouts.

IS RUNNING FOR YOU?

If you do not have any health problems or serious injuries from your walking program and have had difficulty elevating your heart rate to the target level, you may be ready for the walk-run-walk program. Your walking workouts may have improved your fitness, but most likely you have not reached your physiological potential. The only way you can keep improving is to increase your exercise efforts. At this point, running may be the most logical means by which to achieve this.

USING THE WALKING CHARTS

1. *Warm-up with slow and easy walking* for three or four minutes, then do the stretching exercises. (Fitness 12) to loosen and tone your major muscle groups. A cool-down period for five to six minutes is equally important.

2. *For your main conditioning session,* walk briskly for the designated time or distance listed in the charts.

3. *After 10 minutes of walking, stop and check your pulse rate* for 10 seconds and check it again at the end of your walk. Try to walk fast enough to keep your pulse rate elevated to or near your target rate.

4. *If you become winded or unusually tired, or if your pulse rate is too rapid* (above your target rate) slow down to a more reasonable walking pace.

5. *The charts are arranged in steps.* A step represents two workouts (one workout per day), the second being a repeat of the first workout in the step. Providing you feel no adverse fatigue an hour after you have repeated the workout on the second day, you can move up to the next step. If your walking bout seems excessive, cut back to the previous step or continue repeating the workout you are on until you respond more favorably.

6. *The charts are designed so you will increase* your walking time four minutes (also your distance) every two days until you can walk for one hour (approximately three miles). Then you are encouraged to walk the same distance faster until you reach an advanced maintenance level.

7. *Once you have walked your way through the starter and intermediate charts,* you may be ready to include some short periods of running into your workout. If so, refer to the next chapter for additional instruction for making this change.

8. *Keep a record.* As you complete each workout session, check the appropriate box on the chart you are following. Also record your heart rate taken immediately at the end of your brisk walking. Keeping an accurate record of your workouts helps you to follow your progress from day to day systematically.

Chart 6-1. Walking—Starter Program

STEP	SESSION	MAXIMAL MET CAPACITY	THE WORKOUT		DISTANCE GOALS (miles)	PEAK TRAINING HEART RATE	GENERAL COMMENTS
			VIGOROUS WALKING (minute)				
1	1 ☐ and 2 ☐	4 or below	15 to 20		.5 to .8		
2	3 ☐ and 4 ☐		20		.9 to 1.0		
3	5 ☐ and 6 ☐	4.5	24		1.1 to 1.2		
4	7 ☐ and 8 ☐		28		1.3 to 1.4		
5	9 ☐ and 10 ☐	5.0	32		1.4 to 1.6		
6	11 ☐ and 12 ☐		36		1.7 to 1.8		
7	13 ☐ and 14 ☐	5.5	40		1.9 to 2.0		
8	15 ☐ and 16 ☐		44		2.1 to 2.2		

Chart 6-2. Walking—Intermediate Program

STEP	SESSION	MAXIMAL MET CAPACITY	THE WORKOUT VIGOROUS WALKING (minute)	DISTANCE GOALS (miles)	PEAK TRAINING HEART RATE	GENERAL COMMENTS
9	17 ☐ and 18 ☐	6	48	2.3 to 2.4		
10	19 ☐ and 20 ☐		52	2.5 to 2.6		
11	21 ☐ and 22 ☐		56	2.7 to 2.8		
12	23 ☐ and 24 ☐		60	2.9 to 3.0		
13	25 ☐ and 26 ☐	6.5	58	3.0		
14	27 ☐ and 28 ☐		56	3.0		
15	29 ☐ and 30 ☐		54	3.0		
16	31 ☐ and 32 ☐		52	3.0		

Chart 6-3. Walking—Advanced Program (Increase Distance)

STEP	SESSION	MAXIMAL MET CAPACITY	THE WORKOUT		PEAK TRAINING HEART RATE	GENERAL COMMENTS
			VIGOROUS WALKING (minute)	DISTANCE GOALS (miles)		
17	33 ☐ and 34 ☐	7	56	3.3 to 3.4		
18	35 ☐ and 36 ☐		60	3.5 to 3.6		
19	37 ☐ and 38 ☐	7.5	64	3.7 to 3.8		
20	39 ☐ and 40 ☐		68	3.9 to 4.0		

7

Running

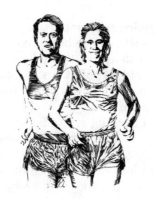

According to a 1986 Gallup poll, approximately 23 million Americans run or jog regularly, not only for maintaining physical fitness but for fun.

In most cases, if you are over 40 and have been inactive in recent years, you should start with the walking charts. After weeks of progressive workouts to the point where you can handle a three-mile walk with ease, then begin the run-walk program.

Running Chart 7-1 has been designed to introduce you gradually to running. At the start, short segments of running are inserted into your walking workouts. Running makes it easier for you to train at your target heart rate (70 percent HR reserve). Eventually you will work up to running two to three miles, four or five times a week. This goal is well within the reach of most people who have no serious health limitations.

Some people only walk for a couple of weeks before they begin running. Others start running and walking right away. Where you start, of course, depends on your initial level of fitness. If you rate low in the initial tests, then your first workouts will involve more walking. Eventually you will be running more and walking less. Keep in mind the basic concept of alternating running and walking—the assurance of completing a certain amount of total work during the exercise session. Exercising at your target heart rate for at least 30 minutes is your goal.

Fitness running can be enjoyable. In addition to the health benefits, people also gain a good feeling from using their bodies in a vigorous manner. Be careful not to overdo it. Injuries, along with disillusionment, may result. Individuals who say running is boring may not have approached running properly. They have experienced crash running programs and expected overnight miraculous results. The following guidelines will help you realize some of the pleasures of running.

WHERE TO RUN

As in walking, it is important to choose a good place to run. Stable and smooth surfaces are best, since rough and uneven surfaces may keep you off balance and could lead to an injury. Avoid heavy automobile traffic and its pollutants. If you have to run where there are cars and trucks, always face oncoming traffic. If you run at night or in the early morning darkness, try to choose a course with street lights. Wear bright-colored clothing and reflective safety gear.

Explore your course by car, if possible, before you run it, to determine the mileage. If you travel, ask others where to run. Running in different cities and towns can be quite interesting.

Indoor tracks are another possibility. Many universities and colleges have indoor tracks opened during certain hours to the public while some health and fitness clubs have small tracks.

WHAT TO WEAR

The late Jim Fixx, in his best-seller *The Complete Book of Running*, observed that "some of the special pleasures (of running) come from being out in weather that drives more faint-hearted people indoors." Many runners enjoy running during supposedly unfavorable weather— falling snow, crisp, cold, clear mornings or gentle rain. As Fixx wrote " . . . there are few conditions under which it is impossible to run in comfort." Obviously, your comfort depends on selecting the right running gear for different types of weather.

Many people tend to overdress for cold weather. Your body generates heat as you exercise, so you need less clothing than normal. Keep your fingers and ears protected from frostbite with a good pair of mittens and a stocking cap. A nylon or cotton/polyester windbreaker, with a full length zipper, is an excellent outer garment. Besides blocking the cold winds, you can take it off when you don't need it and tie it around your waist. One of your layers should be a turtleneck jersey. Just remember to dress so your head and torso are warm.

Can you freeze your lungs while running? The answer is no. Research has shown the air you breathe is adequately warmed before reaching your windpipe and lungs. Heart patients, however, may experience chest pains when breathing cold air and should avoid unnecessary activity in cold temperatures.

In warm weather wear a minimal amount of white or light-colored clothing that reflect the sunlight. Do not wear rubberized jackets or pants to sweat off pounds—you only loose water, not fat. This type of clothing holds the heat in dangerously and can cause serious problems or death. (See Chapter 12).

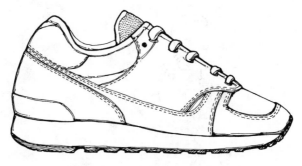

Figure 7-1. Running footgear.

We hope you are not confronted with severe weather conditions when you begin your program. Such conditions can be discouraging. However, as you get in better shape, you will be able to tolerate changing temperatures and weather conditions.

Good footgear is essential (Figure 7-1). Sneakers are too stiff in the forefoot, too low in the heel, and lack good side support for running.

HOW TO RUN

Running, like any physical activity, requires some skill. The repetitive cadence of an experienced runner looks simple and natural. However, the smooth and flowing interaction of the parts of the body while running represents an efficiency of movement for which there is no magic formula. Certain practices can help you improve your running skills.

Maintain proper posture while running. Good posture and running mechanics come from maintaining good muscle tone. Follow the Fitness 12 (see Chapter 5), and focus on the abdominal cruncher or curl and push-ups as presented in Chapter 10. Poor muscle tone leads to sagging bellys and projecting buttocks. Keep your body erect, head up, and shoulders and hips level, with a relaxed arm swing and leg stride. Your foot should fall directly under the body (Figure 7-2).

Avoid a jerky, inefficent style. Experiment until you find your optimal strike length. Run with your toes pointed straight. Avoid excessive bouncing, carrying your arms and hands too high, and swinging your hands across the center line of your body.

Do not run on your toes. Many beginning runners start this way. A heel-to-the-ball or a flat-foot landing are accepted for endurance-type running. These methods provide the maximum amount of shoe surface for landing.

In the flat-foot landing, the entire outside of the sole meets the

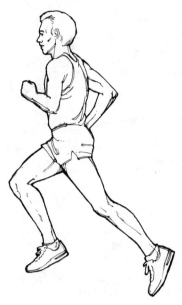

Figure 7-2. Running motion.

ground at one time. The heel-to-the-ball landing is quite similar except you set the outside of your heel down first and roll your weight along the sole and push off with the ball of your foot. You run almost flat-footed, with your heel touching the ground slightly before the ball of your foot.

Some elite distance runners are "mid-foot strikers", because they cover 26 miles at a five-minute mile pace, they find it more efficient to run on the forefoot.

REGULATING YOUR RUNNING INTENSITY

The key to your individualized running program is to discover your own workload intensity, or more specifically, your running pace. The intensity of your running segments should be well within your capabilities, at approximately 70 percent HR reserve. After about five to six minutes of run-walks, check your pulse rate within a few seconds. At the start, it is quite common for people to run too fast, causing the heart rate to rise above the target rate. Eventually you will learn to adjust your pace. Once you find your cruising speed, you will find it easy to stay well within your limits. For most people, the target heart rate is in the neighborhood of 130 to 170 beats per minute. At such a heart rate elevation, you should be able to carry on a conversation with a friend. If you cannot talk, you are probably exercising too intensely. Slow down to a more comfortable pace.

SELECTING A STARTING POINT

The running charts are based on 25 years of actual experience with successful programs involving school children, college students, and adults of all ages. These charts make it easy for you to meet your individual needs regardless of age, sex, or fitness level.

Those who have progressed through the walking charts and are ready to incorporate some running in the workout, begin with running Chart 7-1 on page 95. Those just starting should be sure they can do the three-mile walk test in close to 45 minutes before starting a running program.

Your goal in a few weeks is to complete a run of 10 minutes non-stop at your target heart rate. Eventually your goal will be to sustain a slow run of 20 to 30 minutes without stopping. Under normal circumstances this can be accomplished in 12 to 15 weeks of proper training.

If you stay with the chart's sequences, you will be pleasantly surprised to see how easy it is to progress without injury. Eventually you will realize the good feeling and exuberance that results from running; furthermore, you will enjoy seeing how well your body adapts to each exercise step.

AVOID INJURIES

While running is beneficial, it can cause injuries. Shin splints, knee pain, muscle pulls, tendinitis, and even fractures are common among runners. Fortunately, we know how to prevent many of these problems.

Always stretch before and after your workout. As you increase your capabilities to run longer and farther, you will need to stretch more during your warm-up and cool-down periods. The Fitness 12 or similar stretching and toning exercises must be a regular part of every workout. Although this is sound advice, many people often cut down or even refrain from doing any stretching. However, those who have suffered from various running-related injuries know the importance of warming up and cooling down.

Many running injuries are the result of overuse—doing too much, too soon. Therefore, follow the recommended charts, especially if you are beginning. Your body needs time to adjust. Following the systematic plan of increased workloads will help.

Expect some soreness of muscles and joints during the first few weeks. These discomforts are due to new demands on your muscles, even if you have been walking for eight to 10 weeks. Each activity involves a specific set of muscle groups. This initial discomfort should not hinder your daily progress. Eventually the soreness will disappear. However, it may reappear as you speed up your program, add another exercise, or change to another sport or activity.

Use your heart-rate response as a gauge of your intensity. Learn to anticipate and recognize signs of fatigue and exhaustion. Remember, rhythmic endurance-type exercise should lead to a state of mental and physical harmony; although somewhat taxing, no workout should be a torture.

THE RUNNING CHARTS

The running charts (pages 95–102) consist of systematically arranged workouts to assist you in running continuously for 20 minutes within a period of 15 weeks. Chart 7-1 is the starter program—it goes for 20 sessions or about five weeks. After warming up, your main workout consists of walking briskly for a designated time before beginning the run-walk segment of your workout. The importance of preceding your running segments with brisk walks must be emphasized. This approach has proved helpful in avoiding injuries during the early stages.

After completing step 10 of the first chart, you will be running a total distance of about one mile. Chart 7-2, covering an additional five weeks, takes you to the point where your total running distance reaches two miles. Then you are ready for Chart 7-3. This brings you to the point where you can run and walk continuously for 20 minutes or approximately two miles. The box on page 94 outlines how to use these charts. Remember to begin each session with warm-up stretching exercises. After you complete each workout, cool down with slow walking and stretching exercises of the large leg muscles.

There are 10 steps in each chart, and each step calls for repeating the same workout the next session. Each run-walk workout is preceded by some walking followed by alternating short segments of running and brisk walking. When the run-walk segments are completed, a period of brisk walking is called for. As you advance through each step, the time for each running segment is increased. Also, the number of sets of run-walks are planned so that each workout requires a little more total work than the previous step. Some of the early steps in Chart 7-1 are arranged so you will do considerably more walking (up to as much as one mile) before beginning any run-walk sets.

The first three charts give no reference to distance. When beginning runners become preoccupied with distance, they are more apt to run too fast. Go easy enough to carry on a conversation. Your aim is to challenge your heart, lungs, and muscles vigorously but well within your capabilities. Also, it is important to spread your vigorous exercise over 30 minutes or so.

As you progress through the charts, you will be sustaining your running longer. Eventually you'll be able to run comfortably for 20 minutes non-stop (see Chart 7-3). In terms of distance, this will be anywhere from 1 ¾ to 2 miles, depending on your running speed.

Now you are probably ready to think distance. Chart 7-4 helps you realize the goal of running continuously for three miles (or 30 minutes) at your target heart rate. This chart has worked well for many people. If you want to strive for additional mileage, up to as much as six miles or more, you should progress slowly. Do not increase your total weekly mileage more than one or two miles.

Be sure to walk briskly when the charts call for walking, even between your running segments. And don't overlook the importance of these walking segments between each run. A general rule: as your running distance increases, walk longer but do not walk for more than half the time of each preceding run. For example, if you run for two minutes, then your walking interval should not be longer than one minue.

You are working too hard if you sense an overall body fatigue an hour after you complete one of the workouts. Repeat the same workout until you recover more favorably. If you continue to be overly fatigued after your workouts, try running at a slower pace or move back a step. If this fatigue persists, seek medical counsel. In most instances, if you closely follow these charts you can do a little more every two days. Don't forget—physical fitness is a lifetime pursuit, so start out slowly and progress gradually.

Once you study the charts and understand how to read them, you will find them easy to follow. For example, refer to running Chart 7-1, step 1 (page 95) The workout begins with 20 minutes of brisk walking. Then under the "Run-Walk" heading you will notice it requires running for 30 seconds, followed by brisk walking for 30 seconds. This should be repeated four times, as indicated by the 4X. Then you walk for an additional 10 minutes for a total exercise time of 33.5 minutes. Keep in mind this doesn't include the time for warm-up or the five minutes or so for a cooling down period of slow walking and some stretching.

When you reach Chart 7-3, you are getting close to the point where you will be able to sustain 10- and 20-minute running sessions. In steps 8 and 9 you are getting to the point where you can run a mile without stopping. For most individuals this represents a day of great accomplishment—it was worth all your efforts.

Chart 7-4 gives you the guidelines for increasing your run to three or more miles. Running for 20 to 30 minutes on a regular basis will help you maintain a healthy and physically fit body. You have embarked on a lifetime program. It took time, energy, and effort to reach your goal. From this point on, it is easier to maintain it.

USING THE RUNNING CHARTS

1. *Warm up with slow and easy walking* for three to four minutes, then do the stretching exercises (Fitness 12) to loosen and tone your major muscles groups. Likewise, a cool-down period of walking and stretching is equally important for five to six minutes.

2. *For your main workout,* walk briskly for the designated time listed in the charts before undertaking the run-walk bouts. This part of your workout is very important in helping you avoid injuries that are common during early stages of most running programs.

3. *After you have completed a few of the run-walks,* check your pulse rate for 10 seconds as you complete a run. You should be near your target heart rate.

4. *If your pulse rate is too rapid (above your target rate),* slow down. You should be able to carry on a conversation as you run.

5. *The charts are arranged in steps.* A step represents two workouts, the second being a repeat of the first workout in the step.

6. *If your main workout of walking and run-walks* seems excessive, cut back on your running pace or move back a step until you respond more favorably.

7. *The charts are designed so you will systematically* increase your total work output every two days until you can sustain continuous running for 20 to 30 minutes. Then you are ready to consider runs of longer duration.

8. *Keep a record.* As you complete each workout session, make a check in the appropriate box on the chart you are following. Also record your heart rate taken at the end of your last vigorous running bout. Keeping an accurate record of your workouts helps you stay with it and enables you to systematically follow your progress from day to day.

Chart 7-1. Run-Walk

THE WORKOUT

STEP	SESSION	MAXI-MAL MET CAPAC-ITY	BRISK WALKING (min.)	RUN-WALKS	BRISK WALK-ING (min.)	TOTAL WORK-OUT TIME (min.)	PEAK TRAIN-ING HEART RATE	GENERAL COMMENTS
1	1 ☐ and 2 ☐	8	20	run 30 sec. and walk 30 sec. (4X)	10	33.5		
2	3 ☐ and 4 ☐		17.5	run 30 sec. and walk 30 sec. (6X)	10	33.0		
3	5 ☐ and 6 ☐		15	run 30 sec. and walk 30 sec. (6X) then run 45. sec. and walk 40 sec. (2X)	8	31.0		
4	7 ☐ and 8 ☐		15	run 45 sec. and walk 30 sec. (4X) then run 1 min. and walk 30 sec. (2X)	8	30.5		
5	9 ☐ and 10☐		12	run 45 sec. and walk 30 sec. (4X) then run 1 min. and walk 30 sec. (3X)	8	29.0		
6	11 ☐ and 12 ☐	8.5	12	run 45 sec. and walk 30 sec. (4X) then run 1 min. and walk 30 sec. (4X)	8	30.5		
7	13 ☐ and 14 ☐		10	run 45 sec. and walk 30 sec. (2X) then run 1 min. and walk 30 sec. (5X)	6	27.0		
8	15 ☐ and 16 ☐		10	run 45 sec. and walk 30 sec. (2X) then run 1 min. and walk 30 sec. (6X)	6	29.5		

Chart 7-1. Cont.

			THE WORKOUT				
STEP	SESSION	MAXI-MAL MET CAPAC-ITY	BRISK WALKING (min.)	RUN-WALKS	BRISK WALK-ING (min.)	TOTAL WORK-OUT TIME (min.)	PEAK TRAIN-ING HEART RATE	GENERAL COMMENTS
9	17 ☐ and 18 ☐	8.5	10	run 45 sec. and walk 30 sec. (2X) then run 1 min. and walk 30 sec. (7X)	6	30.0		
10	19 ☐ and 20 ☐		10	run 45 sec. and walk 30 sec. (2X) then run 1 min. and walk 30 sec. (8X)	6	31.5		

Chart 7-2. Run-Walk

STEP	SESSION	MAXI-MAL CAPAC-ITY	THE WORKOUT			TOTAL WORK-OUT TIME (min.)	PEAK TRAIN-ING HEART RATE	GENERAL COMMENTS
			BRISK WALKING (min.)	RUN-WALKS	BRISK WALK-ING (min.)			
1	1 ☐ and 2 ☐	9	10	run 1 min. and walk 30 sec. (8X) then run 1.5 min. and walk 45 sec. (2X)	4	28		
2	3 ☐ and 4 ☐		10	run 1 min. and walk 30 sec. (6X) then run 1.5 min. and walk 45 sec. (4X)	4	28		
3	5 ☐ and 6 ☐		8	run 1 min. and walk 30 sec. (5X) then run 1.5 min. and walk 45 sec. (4X) run 2 min. (1X)	4	30		
4	7 ☐ and 8 ☐		8	run 1 min. and walk 30 sec. (2X) then run 1.5 min. and walk 45 sec. (6X) run 2 min. and walk 1 min. (2X)	4	32		
5	9 ☐ and 10☐		6	run 1 min. and walk 30 sec. (2X) then run 1.5 min. and walk 45 sec. (4X) run 2 min. and walk 1 min. (4X)	4	33		
6	11 ☐ and 12 ☐	9.5	6	run 1 min. and walk 30 sec. (2X) then run 1.5 min. and walk 45 sec. (2X) run 2 min. and walk 1 min. (6X)	4	33		

Chart 7-2. Cont.

STEP	SESSION	MAXI-MAL CAPAC-ITY	BRISK WALKING (min.)	THE WORKOUT RUN-WALKS	BRISK WALK-ING (min.)	TOTAL WORK-OUT TIME (min.)	PEAK TRAIN-ING HEART RATE	GENERAL COMMENTS
7	13 ☐ and 14 ☐		4	run 1.5 min. and walk 30 sec. (2X) then run 2 min. and walk 45 sec. (8X)	2	32		
8	15 ☐ and 16 ☐		4	run 1.5 min. and walk 30 sec. (2X) then run 2 min. and walk 45 sec. (8X)	2	32		
9	17 ☐ and 18 ☐		2	run 2 min. and walk 30 sec. (8X) then run 3 min. and walk 1 min. (2X)	2	30		
10	19 ☐ and 20 ☐		2	run 2 min. and walk 30 sec. (6X) then run 3 min. and walk 1 min. (4X)	2	34		

Chart 7-3. Run-Walk

STEP	SESSION	MAXIMAL MET CAPACITY	THE WORKOUT		PEAK TRAINING HEART RATE	GENERAL COMMENTS
			RUN-WALKS (Approximately 30 min. per workout)	TOTAL RUNNING TIME (min.)		
1	1 □ and 2 □	10	run 2 min., walk 30 sec. (5X) run 3 min., walk 1 min. (5X)	25		
2	3 □ and 4 □		run 2 min., walk 30 sec. (3X) run 3 min., walk 1 min. (4X) run 4 min., walk 2 min. (2X)	26		
3	5 □ and 6 □		run 3 min., walk 1 min. (4X) run 4 min., walk 2 min. (3X)	24		
4	7 □ and 8 □		run 3 min., walk 1 min. (3X) run 4 min., walk 2 min. (4X)	25		
5	9 □ and 10 □		run 3 min., walk 1 min. (2X) run 4 min., walk 1.5 min. (2X) run 5 min., walk 2 min. (2X)	24		
6	11 □ and 12 □	11	run 4 min., walk 1.5 min. (2X) run 5 min., walk 2 min. (2X) run 6 min. (1X)	24		
7	13 □ and 14 □	11	run 4 min., walk 1 min. (2X) run 8 min., walk 2.5 min. (2X)	24		

Chart 7-3. Cont.

STEP	SESSION	MAXIMAL MET CAPACITY	THE WORKOUT		TOTAL RUNNING TIME (min.)	PEAK TRAINING HEART RATE	GENERAL COMMENTS
			RUN-WALKS (Approximately 30 min. per workout)				
8	15 ☐ and 16 ☐		run 4 min., walk 1 min. (2X) run 10 min., walk 2.5 min. (1X) run 6 min. (1X)		24		
9	17 ☐ and 18 ☐		run 4 min., walk 1 min. (1X) run 10 min., walk 2 min. (2X)		24		
10	19 ☐ and 20 ☐		run 20 min.		20		

Chart 7-4. Run-Walk

STEP	SESSION	MAXIMAL MET CAPACITY	THE WORKOUT RUN-WALKS	TOTAL DISTANCE RUN (miles)	PEAK TRAINING HEART RATE	GENERAL COMMENTS
F I R S T W E E K						
1	Mon.	☐	run 2 mile or for 20 to 24 min. walk 2-4 min. run .5 mile or for 5 to 6 min.	2.5		
2	Tue.	☐	run 1.5 mile or 15 to 18 min. walk 2 min. run 1.0 mile or 10 to 12 min.	2.5		
3	Thur.	☐	run 2.5 mile or 25 to 30 min.	2.5		
4	Fri.	☐	run 1.5 mile or 15 to 18 min.	1.5		
S E C O N D W E E K						
5	Mon.	☐	run 2.0 mile or for 20 to 24 min. walk 2-4 min. run .5 mile or for 5 to 6 min. walk 1 min. run .5 mile or for 5 to 6 min.	2.0		
6	Tue.	☐	run 1.5 mile or 15 to 18 min. walk 2-3 min. run 1.5 mile or 15 to 18 min.	3.0		
7	Thur.	☐	run 3 mile or for 30 to 36 min.	3.0		
8	Fri.	☐	run 2.5 mile or for 25 to 30 min.	2.5		

Chart 7-4. Cont.

STEP		SESSION	MAXIMAL MET CAPACITY	THE WORKOUT	TOTAL DISTANCE RUN (miles)	PEAK TRAINING HEART RATE	GENERAL COMMENTS
				RUN-WALKS			
T H I R D	9	Mon. ☐		run 2.5 mile or for 25 to 30 min. walk 2-4 min. run 1.0 mile or for 10 to 12 min.	3.5		
	10	Tue. ☐		run 2.0 mile or 20 to 24 min. walk 2-3 min. run 1.5 mile or 15 to 18 min.	3.5		
W E E K	11	Thur. ☐		run 3.5 mile or for 35 to 42 min.	3.5		
	12	Fri. ☐		run 3 mile or for 30 to 36 min.	3.0		

8

Swimming

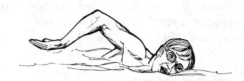

Swimming, considered one of the best forms of exercise, involves all the major muscles in your body. As a result, it gives you more of a total conditioning effect than many other sports. Besides being an excellent means for developing cardiorespiratory fitness, it can be refreshing. The rhythmic movements of the muscles of the arms, legs, and trunk and the stimulation of the cool water are highly beneficial to blood flow and muscle stimulation. The buoying effect of the water in a non-weight-bearing position reduces excessive pressure on the joints and bones. Swimmers are less susceptible to the muscle soreness and tightness common to runners or the shin splints, tennis elbow, or torn ligaments seen in other sports.

Swimming has its drawbacks. You must know how to swim. Swimming instruction is available at private clubs and fitness or recreation centers. Even if you are not a good swimmer at the start, you can carry out a productive conditioning workout in the water. As you improve your skills, you can fully realize not only the conditioning benefits of endurance swimming but the satisfaction of moving effectively in the water.

Another drawback is the availability of a pool. It is necessary to swim without interruption in an open lane. Fortunately more pool directors are setting aside certain hours for lap swimming.

To obtain maximum benefits from a swimming workout, you must be stroking at a cadence that adequately challenges your heart, lungs, and muscles. Just as in running and brisk walking, your heart rate elevation is the key factor for regulating the intensity of your workout. Stroking must be vigorous enough to elevate your heart rate to your 70 percent HR reserve level.

Research shows that swimming at a low level of intensity is quite easy. Individuals who have good swimming skills and high body fat percentages can swim continuously without much effort. Unfortunately, they do not make reasonable improvements in their fitness measurements. Swimming for these people can be compared to a leisurely bike ride or a stroll. The workouts are not sufficiently intense to produce a training effect.

WHERE TO SWIM

To swim for fitness, you need a pool or body of water with marked lanes. Many fitness centers have specific times for fitness training. The membership fee may be worth the convenience. If you live near a college or university, check on the availability of their pools. Many set aside lanes for fitness swimming during off hours and offer instruction to the public.

A certified lifeguard should be on duty during swimming sessions. If you swim in a private home pool make certain there is someone with you. Never swim alone.

Most pools are 25 yards long; some are measured in meters. In this book, a lap refers to the length of the pool or 25 yards. If you use pools of different lengths, modify the instructions in the charts.

WHAT TO WEAR

Besides a proper swimsuit, you only need a pair of swimming goggles to protect your eyes from chlorine and other chemicals. Be sure they fit you properly and do not leak. Some people like to swim with bathing caps. Again, select one that does not leak.

Accessory items might include a kickboard for kicking drills or small pulling tubes to wrap around your ankles for drag in the water. (Competitive swimmers call them pulling drills.) Most pools have these accessories on hand.

SELECTING A STARTING POINT

Why do you want to swim? Perhaps your intent is to use swimming as a complement to running or walking. Others suffer joint problems and are unable to run. Regardless of the reason, some preliminary considerations are in order before you plunge into the pool.

How do you determine your starting point for swimming? If you can swim, but have not been in the pool in recent years, start with swimming Chart 8-1. If you have been walking, running, or cycling on a regular basis and want to start swimming, you should not have to start at the beginning with the swimming charts. You may be able to progress more rapidly through the swimming charts. Just don't overdo it!

HOW TO SWIM FOR FITNESS

If you are not a very good swimmer, the distance of a lap looks endless. If you are going to use swimming as a main part of your fitness training, it is wise to seek ways to refine your techniques. The front crawl stroke (Figure 8-1) is the most common stroke for fitness training. Nevertheless, to add variety to your workouts with segments of easier swimming, learn the backstroke, sidestroke, and the breaststroke. Even if you are a good swimmer, try to improve your techniques. Efficient swimming seldom comes naturally. You need to devote time to mastery of most swimming skills.

REGULATING YOUR SWIMMING INTENSITY

Swimming becomes a training exercise when it is done at a challenging intensity. Don't worry about how far you can swim continuously. Instead, move at a speed vigorous enough to elevate your heart rate to your target level. Your eventual goal will be to swim continuously for 30 minutes or more.

As in walking and running, it is important to warm up properly using the stretching and toning exercises described in Chapter 5.

At first, think in terms of swimming one lap at a time. For example, in Chart 8-1, step 1, swim one lap, then rest 15 to 30 seconds. Repeat this

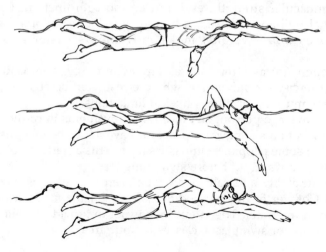

Figure 8-1. Front crawl stroke.

sequence eight times. Once you handle this goal, go to the next step, which calls for adding two laps. When you can do 12 one-lappers alternated with periods of short rest, you are ready to start including some two-lappers in your workout (see Chart 8-2, page 109). Don't worry about speed. Find a rhythmical pace that you can maintain reasonably well for the prescribed distance—whether it is one lap or four. Many pools designate lanes for slower swimmers to keep other lanes open for the faster paced swimmers.

Be sure to check your heart rate halfway through your workout and at the end. Many pools have a continuously running clock, often called a pace clock. It has a huge second hand to help swimmers keep time of laps and rest periods and to check pulse rates. Eventually you will determine the effort it takes to provide a suitable stimulus to your heart eliminating the need to check each day.

It may take several weeks or months before you can swim for 30 to 40 minutes without stopping. However, by following the swimming charts through chart 8-5 you will soon be swimming more total laps, swimming more laps continuously, and getting stronger. Remember the basic rule! Your workout should always be set so you feel fully recovered and rested within an hour of its completion.

SWIMNASTICS

Swimnastics refers to activities and exercise performed while the body is submerged in water. The President's Council on Physical Fitness and Sports has coined the term Aqua-Dynamics to describe such programs. Specific exercises and routines are carried out in the water to enhance muscular strength, endurance, and coordination. Reduced gravitational pull and the water's buoyancy (which supports the body and reduces body weight) make movements easier and more comfortable.

Although not as strenuous as lap-swimming, swimnastics is a means of exercise for individuals who are restricted because of painful joints, weak muscles, or other physical limitations.

For the average person, significant improvements in cardiorespiratory fitness from a swimnastics program have yet to be demonstrated. However, for some people, swimnastics represents a starting point or an effective way to warm up before swimming laps.

Many flexibility and calisthenic-type exercises, such as those presented in Chapter 5, can be modified so reasonable facsimiles can be performed in the water. The intent here is not to provide a swimnastics routine. Check for swimnastic classes in your area.

USING THE SWIMMING CHARTS

1. *Start out by warming up* with some stretching exercises. Use this period for loosening and activating your major muscle groups. When your main conditioning segment is complete, repeat some of these exercises during your cool-down.

2. *The swimming charts provide* a systematic pattern of steps designed so you will increase your swimming time and distance in a graduated manner every two days.

3. *The charts are arranged in steps.* A step represents two workouts, the second being a repeat of the first workout in the step.

4. *If you feel no adverse fatigue* one hour after you have repeated a workout for the second day, move up to the next step. If your swimming segments seem excessive, cut back to the previous step or continue repeating the step you are on until you respond more favorably.

5. *If you do not recover reasonably well,* take a longer rest before swimming your next segment during the suggested time period of rest.

6. *At the end of each chart you should* swim the designated distance as continuously as possible with rest periods when you wish.

7. *Once you have swum your way through the charts,* you are ready to extend your workouts to include more continuous swimming. Your ultimate goal is to be able to swim continuously (without a rest period) a half-mile (880 yards) or more.

8. *Keep a record.* As you complete each workout session check the appropriate box on the chart you are following. Record the heart rate taken at the end of your last vigorous swimming lap. Keeping an accurate record of your workouts helps you stay with it and enables you to follow your progress from day to day.

Chart 8-1. Swimming (Swim-Rest)

STEP	SESSION	THE WORKOUT SWIM-REST (lengths)	TOTAL WORK-OUT TIME (min.)	APPROXI-MATE TOTAL DISTANCE SWAM (yd.)	TRAIN-ING HEART RATE	GENERAL COMMENTS
1	1 ☐ and 2 ☐	Swim 1 lap, rest 15 to 30 sec. (8X)	12-20	200		
4	7 ☐ and 8 ☐	Swim 1 lap, rest 15 to 30 sec. (10X)	16-24	250		
5	9 ☐ and 10 ☐	Swim 1 lap, rest 15 to 30 sec. (12X)	20-28	300		
6	11 ☐ and 12 ☐	Swim a total of 12 laps, rest when needed but no longer than 15 to 30 sec.	20-30	300		

Chart 8-2. Swimming (Swim-Rest)

STEP	SESSION	THE WORKOUT SWIM-REST	TOTAL WORK-OUT TIME (min.)	APPROXI-MATE TOTAL DISTANCE SWAM (yd.)	TRAIN-ING HEART RATE	GENERAL COMMENTS
1	1 ☐ and 2 ☐	Swim 1 lap, rest 15 to 30 sec. (10X) Swim 2 laps, rest 45 sec. (2X)	24 to 28	350		
2	3 ☐ and 4 ☐	Swim 1 lap, rest 15 to 30 sec. (8X) Swim 2 laps, rest 45 sec. (4X)	24 to 28	400		
3	5 ☐ and 6 ☐	Swim 1 lap, rest 15 to 30 sec. (6X) Swim 2 laps, rest 45 sec. (6X)	24 to 30	450		
4	7 ☐ and 8 ☐	Swim 1 lap, rest 15 to 20 sec. (4X) Swim 2 laps, rest 45 sec. (8X)	24 to 30	500		
5	9 ☐ and 10 ☐	Swim 1 lap, rest 15 sec. (2X) Swim 2 laps, rest 30 to 45 sec.	24 to 30	550		
6	11 ☐ and 12 ☐	Swim a total of 24 laps, resting when needed but no longer than 15 to 30 sec.	24 to 35	600		

Chart 8-3. Swimming (Swim-Rest)

STEP	SESSION	THE WORKOUT SWIM-REST	TOTAL WORK-OUT TIME (min.)	APPROXI-MATE TOTAL DISTANCE SWAM (yd.)	TRAIN-ING HEART RATE	GENERAL COMMENTS
1	1 ☐ and 2 ☐	Swim 2 laps, rest 20 to 30 sec. (10X) Swim 3 laps, rest 30 sec. (2X)	22 to 30	650		
2	3 ☐ and 4 ☐	Swim 2 laps, rest 20 sec. (8X) Swim 3 laps, rest 30 sec. (4X)	24 to 32	700		
3	5 ☐ and 6 ☐	Swim 2 laps, rest 20 sec. (6X) Swim 3 laps, rest 30 sec. (6X)	26 to 36	750		
4	7 ☐ and 8 ☐	Swim 2 laps, rest 10 sec. (4X) Swim 3 laps, rest 20 to 30 sec. (8X)	28 to 36	800		
5	9 ☐ and 10 ☐	Swim 2 laps, rest 10 sec. (2X) Swim 3 laps, rest 20 to 30 sec. (10X)	30 to 38	850		
6	11 ☐ and 12 ☐	Swim a total of 34 laps, rest when needed but no longer than 20 to 30 sec.	24 to 40	850		

Chart 8-4. Swimming (Swim-Rest)

STEP	SESSION	THE WORKOUT SWIM-REST	TOTAL WORK-OUT TIME (min.)	APPROXI-MATE TOTAL DISTANCE SWAM (yd.)	TRAIN-ING HEART RATE	GENERAL COMMENTS
1	1 ☐ and 2 ☐	Swim 3 laps, rest 20 sec. (9X) Swim 4 laps, rest 30 sec. (2X)	28 to 34	825		
2	3 ☐ and 4 ☐	Swim 3 laps, rest 20 sec. (8X) Swim 4 laps, rest 30 sec. (3X)	28 to 34	950		
3	5 ☐ and 6 ☐	Swim 3 laps, rest 20 sec. (7X) Swim 4 laps, rest 30 sec. (4X)	28 to 35	925		
4	7 ☐ and 8 ☐	Swim 3 laps, rest 10 sec. (6X) Swim 4 laps, rest 20 to 30 sec. (5X)	28 to 35	950		
5	9 ☐ and 10 ☐	Swim 3 laps, rest 10 sec. (5X) Swim 4 laps, rest 20 to 30 sec. (6X)	28 to 36	975		
6	11 ☐ and 12 ☐	Swim a total of 40 laps, rest when needed but no longer than 20 to 30 sec.	30 to 40	1000		

Chart 8-5. Swimming (Swim-Rest)

	THE WORKOUT				
STEP	SESSION	SWIM-REST	TOTAL WORK-OUT TIME (min.)	APPROXI-MATE TOTAL DISTANCE SWAM (yd.)	TRAIN-ING HEART RATE	GENERAL COMMENTS
1	1 ☐ and 2 ☐	Swim 4 laps, rest 20 to 30 sec. (6X) Swim 6 laps, rest 30 sec. (3X)	30 to 38	1050		
2	3 ☐ and 4 ☐	Swim 4 laps, rest 20 sec. (5X) Swim 6 laps, rest 30 sec. (4X)	30 to 38	1100		
3	5 ☐ and 6 ☐	Swim 4 laps, rest 20 sec. (4X) Swim 6 laps, rest 20 to 30 sec. (5X)	32 to 40	1250		
4	7 ☐ and 8 ☐	Swim 4 laps, rest 10 sec. (3X) Swim 6 laps, rest 20 sec. (6X)	34 to 42	1400		
5	9 ☐ and 10 ☐	Swim 4 laps, rest 10 sec. (2X) Swim 6 laps, rest 10 to 20 sec. (7X)	36 to 44	1550		
6	11 ☐ and 12 ☐	Swim a total of 64 laps, rest when needed but no longer than 20 to 30 sec.	40 to 48	1600		

9

Bicycling

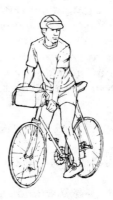

A bicycle is a weekend plaything for some, but for others it provides a main means for keeping in good shape. Many individuals use bicycling as an alternative to running because its cardiorespiratory benefits can equal those of running.

Bicycling for physical fitness requires more exertion than that needed to pedal to the grocery. Leisurely pedaling will not benefit your fitness. However, vigorous, sustained pedaling (within your abilities) can stimulate your lungs, heart, and muscles adequately for improvements. Naturally, the pace at which you ride, just as in walking and running, will govern the fitness benefits of cycling. In general, riding at a pace of four to five minutes a mile (12 to 15 mph), for 30 to 60 minutes, provides an adequate training stimulus for the cardiorespiratory system (70 percent HR reserve).

SELECTING A BIKE

Whether you decide on a 3-or 10-speed bicycle, the bike must be in good mechanical condition. More than a million people are injured in bicycle accidents each year, and some 1,000 die. Many of these accidents are caused by faulty equipment. Bicycles marketed today must meet rigid standards set by the U.S. Consumer Product Safety Commission.

If you become a serious cyclist, a 10-speed bicycle is more practical than a 3-speed. If all you ever plan to do is ride around the block on level terrain, you probably don't need 10 gears. But, if you are interested in going appreciable distances over varying terrain in order to develop and maintain a good level of physical fitness, you should consider a 10-speed.

Make certain your bicycle is adjusted properly for your body. Saddle height, handlebar height, frame size, and stem length are important. An improperly fitted bike can cause muscle and joint strains.

Covering all the ins and outs of selecting and fitting a bike is a chapter in itself. If you are purchasing a bike for the first time, go to a shop specializing in bicycles—one that sells as well as repairs. Proprietors are well trained to fit you properly and keep the bike in good condition.

HOW TO BIKE AND WHERE

It takes skill and savvy to ride a bicycle effectively, especially a 10-speed. Experience will enable you to control your bike under any circumstances. Develop an awareness of road conditions and a realization of your limitations and those of your equipment. Avoid heavy traffic and steep, winding roads until you are a seasoned cyclist.

Learn to anticipate trouble. Be alert for potholes. Hitting one could catapult you into the path of a car. You want to maximize your time achieving your target heart rate, not dodging potholes and traffic. Use common sense in choosing your cycle path. If your community has cycling paths, use them. Being concerned about finding a safe place to bike cannot be overemphasized.

WHAT TO WEAR

Improper clothing can be a hindrance as well as a source of discomfort during your workout. Street clothes are too confining for efficient and enjoyable cycling. Well-designed cycling clothes are light-weight, streamlined, unrestricting, protective, and durable. The items you need depend on how far you travel, frequency, climatic conditions, your level of participation and, of course, your budget.

Your first purchase should be a cycling helmet. Protective headgear has saved many cyclists from serious injury. Choose a lightweight and well-ventilated helmet with a sturdy chin strap. Also, cycling gloves with added padding are essential and offer great protection in a crash or fall.

Many cyclists advocate cycling shoes with stiff shanks. As with running shoes, try on several pairs to get a feel for performance. Toe clips will make you a more efficient rider. The toe clip is a strong, spring-steel fixture bolted to the front side of each pedal with a leather top strap and buckle. It is designed to provide a fixed position for the foot.

AVOIDING INJURIES

The most serious problem any cyclist faces is a fall or collision. You can avoid serious skin abrasions by keeping your arms and legs covered. Some of the new materials are comfortable for year round wear. Always wear a helmet.

Pain commonly comes from a bad riding position. Try to make some adjustments on the bike; adjust the seat or handlebars. Saddle soreness can result from improper seat height. The material in your cycling pants can either cause or prevent minor irritations, boils, and blisters.

Incorrect placement of the feet on the pedals and the distribution of force during the pedaling motion may cause painful joints. Wearing proper footwear is crucial if you are to achieve pain-free cycling.

SELECTING A STARTING POINT

The ultimate aim of a cycling fitness program is to pump your legs at a rate sufficient to adequately challenge your cardiorespiratory system for 30 to 60 minutes. Your first few weeks of training should consist of a moderate riding pace so your leg muscles and body can adjust to the new stresses. Even if you have been running or walking, start with a moderate training plan. You need to prepare your leg and thigh muscles for cycling. Remember, doing too much too soon can lead to fatigue and injuries.

You want to reach the point where you will be able to sustain a continuous ride for 30 minutes. Such an effort is comparable to walking briskly for an hour. Once this is accomplished, you are ready to begin a more vigorous training regimen aimed at helping you reach your fitness potential.

REGULATING YOUR CYCLING INTENSITY

To achieve a training effect with a bicycle, you must cycle almost twice as fast as you would run. Because of the smaller muscle mass used in cycling, the oxygen uptake may be a little less than in running for the same heart rate. The key is to develop the ability to pedal vigorously enough to stress the heart and lungs for a training effect.

You may wonder what pedaling gear you should use to attain a training effect. Most people make the mistake of pedaling in too high a gear. It is better to ride in a lower gear at a higher revolution per minute (rpm) rather than in a higher gear at a lower rpm. As a rule of thumb, spinning at 80 rpm in a gear that can be sustained reasonably well seems to work best.

If you have been inactive in recent months, your first riding workouts should be at a relatively low or moderate speed. Start out by riding for 15 to 20 minutes. Repeat the next day, and then if you recover well within an hour after your riding bout, increase your ride the next day by five minutes. Gradually build up your time until you can ride for 30 minutes non-stop.

THE CYCLING CHARTS

When you can ride for 30 minutes continuously, you are ready to refer to Chart 9-1, on page 118. This sequence provides a simple approach for intensifying your cycling effort. The key is to find the speed and gear at which you can maintain your training heart rate intensity and then use that pedaling speed. Follow the pattern of increasing your number of sets with each step.

After you try out the suggested sets, you may need to adjust the cycling speed to provide a lesser or greater heart rate stimulus. Chart 9-2 provides steps for improving your fitness level. Eventually you will have achieved an endurance base and will be able to ride nine miles or more at your target heart rate.

Once you are in good shape and have mastered the skill of bicycling, you may want to consider longer trips. Long distance touring (50 to 100 miles a day) is becoming a popular pastime during vacations or on weekends.

Develop the habit of keeping a log of your cycling workouts. It can assist you in understanding your responses to exertion and can also be motivating. Note your pulse rate in the early stages. As your pulse levels off, it becomes less important to check it each day. Under unusual conditions, such as an extremely hot day or a very long ride, note how hard your cardiorespiratory system was taxed.

USING THE CYCLING CHARTS

1. *Warm up with the stretching exercises* (Fitness 12) to loosen and tone your major muscle groups. In like manner, cool down with some stretching exercises for about five to six minutes following your main cycling workout.

2. *For those who have been inactive* or who tested at a low-fitness level, your first two to three weeks of riding should be at moderate to low speeds with a gradual build-up of total distance each session. Start with bike rides of just 10 to 15 minutes. Gradually increase your time until you are capable of sustaining a comfortable and continuous ride of 30 minutes.

3. *When you can comfortably ride for 30 minutes* at a low speed, you are ready to begin with Chart 9-1, which calls for a more vigorous intensity.

4. *The charts are arranged in steps.* A step represents two workouts, the second being a repeat of the first workout in that step. If you feel no adverse fatigue one hour after you have repeated the workout on the second day, move to the next step. If your cycling workout seems excessive, cut back to the previous step or continue repeating the workout you are on until you respond more favorably.

5. *The charts are designed so you will systematically* increase your number of cycling sets at your target heart rate. Start with three-minute rides with intermittent one-minute periods of easy cycling, with six repeats (step 1), and progress to four minutes and again strive to reach eight repeats. Remember not to fall into the trap of trying to increase your vigorous cycling workouts faster than the charts prescribe.

6. *As you progress through the charts,* you will reach the point where you can ride for 10 minutes or more at your target heart rate intensity interspersed with short rest periods or easy pedaling.

7. *The charts are based on riding at a six-minute-mile pace (10 mph).* For some, this pace may not be adequate to elevate the heart rate to the target level. It is not uncommon to be able to work comfortably at your target heart rate at speeds closer to 3.5-to 5-minute-mile pace (12 to 17 mph). As you adapt you should be able to ride faster and cover a greater total distance.

8. *You will note that the approximate workout time* ranges from 24 minutes to over 50 minutes of cycling. This amount of time is necessary if you are to achieve training changes comparable to running.

9. *Keep a record.* As you complete each workout session, check the appropriate box on the chart you are following. Also record your heart rate taken at the end of your last vigorous cycling set. Keeping an accurate record of your workouts helps you stay with it, and enables you to systematically follow your progress from day to day.

Chart 9-1. Bicycle Repeats

STEP	SESSION	MAXIMAL MET CAPACITY	THE WORKOUT VIGOROUS/ SLOW CYCLING BOUTS	APPROXIMATE WORKOUT TIME (min.)	APPROXIMATE* DISTANCE OF VIGOROUS CYCLING (miles)	PEAK TRAINING HEART RATE	GENERAL COMMENTS
1	1 ☐ and 2 ☐	7	Cycle 3 min. at THR, then cycle easy or rest 1 min. (6X)	24	3.0		
2	3 ☐ and 4 ☐		Cycle 3 min. at THR, then cycle easy or rest 1 min. (7X)	28	3.5		
3	5 ☐ and 6 ☐	7.5	Cycle 3 min. at THR, then cycle easy or rest 1 min. (8X)	32	4.0		
4	7 ☐ and 8 ☐		Cycle 4 min. at THR, then cycle easy or rest 1 min. (6X)	30	2⅔		
5	9 ☐ and 10 ☐	8	Cycle 4 min. at THR, then cycle easy or rest 1 min. (7X)	35	3⅓		
6	11 ☐ and 12 ☐		Cycle 4 min. at THR, then cycle easy or rest 1 min. (8X)	40	4.0		
7	13 ☐ and 14 ☐	8.5	Cycle 5 min. at THR, then cycle easy or rest 1 min. (6X)	36	5.0		

8	15 ☐ and 16 ☐		Cycle 5 min. at THR, then cycle easy or rest 1 min. (7X)	42	6.0
9	17 ☐ and 18 ☐	9	Cycle 5 min. at THR, then cycle easy or rest 1 min. (8X)	48	6.5
10	19 ☐ and 20 ☐		Cycle for 10 to 12 min. at THR, then cycle easy for 2 min. (3X)	36	6.0

*Actual distance will depend on your cycling speed. The mileage estimated is based on a six-minute-mile (10 mph) pace. Some people may need to ride faster to achieve their target heart rate.

Chart 9-2. Bicycling Repeats

STEP	SESSION	MAXIMAL MET CAPACITY	THE WORKOUT VIGOROUS/ SLOW CYCLING BOUTS	APPROXIMATE WORKOUT TIME (min.)	APPROXIMATE* DISTANCE OF VIGOROUS CYCLING (miles)	PEAK TRAINING HEART RATE	GENERAL COMMENTS
1	1 ☐ and 2 ☐	9.5	Cycle 8 min. at THR, cycle easy for 1 min. (3X) Cycle 10 min. at THR (1X)	37	5.5 to 6		
2	3 ☐ and 4 ☐		Cycle 8 min. at THR, cycle easy for 1 min. (2X) Cycle 10 min. at THR, cycle easy for 1 min. (2X)	40	6		
3	5 ☐ and 6 ☐	10.0	Cycle 8 min. at THR, cycle easy for 1 min. (1X) Cycle 10 min. at THR, cycle easy for 1 min. (3X)	42	6 to 6.5		
4	7 ☐ and 8 ☐		Cycle 10 min. at THR, cycle easy for 1 min. (3X) Cycle 12 min. at THR, cycle easy for 1 min. (1X)	45	7		
5	9 ☐ and 10 ☐	10.5	Cycle 12 min. at THR, cycle easy for 1 min. (2X) Cycle 14 min. at THR, cycle (1X)	40	6 to 6.5		

6	11 □ and 12 □		Cycle 12 min. at THR, cycle easy for 1 min. (1X) Cycle 14 min. at THR, cycle easy for 1 min. (2X)	42	6 to 6.5
7	13 □ and 14 □	11.0	Cycle 14 min. at THR, cycle easy for 1 min. (2X) Cycle 16 min. at THR (1X)	46	7 to 7.5
8	15 □ and 16 □		Cycle 14 min. at THR, cycle easy for 1 min. (1X) Cycle 16 min. at THR, cycle easy for 1 min. (2X)	49	7.5 to 8
9	17 □ and 18 □	12.0	Cycle 16 min. at THR, cycle easy for 1 min. (2X) Cycle 18 min. at THR, cycle easy for 1 min. (1X)	53	8 to 8.5
10	19 □ and 20 □		Cycle 18 min. at THR, cycle easy for 1 min. (3X)	57	9

*Actual distance will depend on your cycling speed. The mileage estimated is based on a six-minute-mile (10 mph) pace. Some people may need to ride faster to achieve their target heart rate.

10

Alternative Cardiorespiratory Fitness Activities

Up to now we have dealt extensively with the four basic aerobic activities—walking, running, swimming, and bicycling. There are other forms of fitness activities you may want to consider. We will mention several briefly.

AEROBICS

Jackie Sorensen has been credited with developing "aerobic dance" which involves walking, running, hopping, skipping, and various arm swings and kicking movements to music. Recently, variations of aerobic dance have lead to a variety of activities that are now popularized as "aerobics."

Routines vary and can be geared to the fitness capabilities of the participants. "Non-impact" and "low-impact" are new approaches that lessen the strain on the legs. In low-impact routines, one foot is always on the floor, eliminating the shock of jumping. Non-impact routines reduce the stress even more as neither foot leaves the floor. Participants can work at low, moderate, or high intensity levels to the same music continuously for 35 to 45 minutes. Your instructor will encourage you to monitor your heart rate to ensure you achieve training effects.

A properly planned and choreographed routine can require complete use of every muscle in the body. Good muscle flexibility is involved, and cardiorespiratory benefits are possible. As usual, the intensity, duration, and frequency of the dance periods determine the benefits.

The release of emotional and mental tension through self-expression to music is a bonus. Fortunately, men are now realizing the benefits of aerobics. Many athletes include aerobics in their training regimens.

The popularity of aerobics classes in private and corporate centers is well-established. However, there is a lack of uniformity or safety in these classes. Poor warm-ups, insufficient instruction, harmful routines and movements, and inadequate cool-downs are among the problems. Recently, in the pursuit of uniformity and safety, aerobics associations such as the International Dance and Exercise Association (IDEA) and the Aerobics and Fitness Association of America (AFAA) have recommended guidelines for aerobic dance. Both have developed national certification programs in an attempt to establish levels of instructor standards. Aerobic workshops and a written examination are required. The American College of Sports Medicine (ACSM) has introduced a Exercise Leader/Aerobics Certification program. In addition to an extensive written exam, each candidate must demonstrate various skills in a 90-minute practicum.

It is important to work out on a good, clean floor. Generally today's floors are suspended wood or carpeted floors with thick padding. Most places have mirrors so you can watch yourself do the movements properly.

Probably the most important aspect of any aerobics class is the qualifications of the instructors. Being friendly and nice are not enough. They have to be good. Search for instructors who show you what to do and then make sure you follow their guidance. Instructors should have an upbeat attitude and help to motivate you to keep up your regular workouts. A good instructor will conduct a safe program that uses all the muscles in your body and provides good cardiorespiratory work, strength toning, and flexibility. Above all, it must be enjoyable.

Good programs should also be informative. Your instructor should not only teach you what muscles you are working but how to work them in proper alignment.

As in any fitness activity, you need to wear comfortable clothes. A good pair of aerobics shoes is essential. Look for good shock absorption, lateral support, and shoe stability. The outer sole should be wide enough to create a solid platform for the foot along with a rigid heel counter to hold the foot in place for the vigorous movements. Less important is the style, which unfortunately too often is the main determining factor when people buy shoes.

Working out in an organized aerobic class is not feasible for everyone. Many individuals depend on exercise videos for fitness information. Some authorities have been critical of the leading videos sold today. Many of the videos are made by movie personalities and former athletes and contain misinformation and harmful routines. Some of these celebrities have begun to work closely with qualified experts. As a result we are beginning to see safe aerobic videos.

We advise individuals, when possible, to join programs led by certified instructors. Learn the routines and then, if you want, purchase a tape that has been recommended by your instructor to supplement your regular classes.

ROPE SKIPPING

Many claims, some exaggerated, have been made about jumping rope: "It doesn't cost much," "Anyone can do it," "You can do it anywhere." A most common one—"It can produce the greatest amount of conditioning in the shortest amount of time"—certainly appeals to the person looking for instant fitness. However, current research has refuted the validity of that particular statement. Skipping rope is good for agility and coordination. However, rope skipping for fitness has to be vigorous. For the highly skilled "rope skipper", studies show the energy expended is quite low. For the unskilled, the workout can be sufficiently stimulating, but no more so than running.

Jumping rope places sudden and rigorous demands on the ankle, knee, and hip joints. This could lead to injury if some precautions are not heeded. Even people who can run for 30 minutes have difficulty jumping for 10 minutes because of the constant force on the legs. Wearing sturdy athletic shoes is imperative.

Like any aerobic exercise, it takes time to achieve optimal benefits. For rope skipping to be an effective mode of fitness training, you must work at a substantial intensity, sustain this intensity long enough, and do it regularly.

If you want to try skipping as a means of training, you need a good rope. It should be long enough to reach from armpit to armpit while passing under both feet. The models with plastic disks that slide around the rope provide a good balance and weight to the rope. Reasonably weighted handles keep the rope from getting tangled.

If you haven't skipped before, you need to learn how to turn the rope, to jump rhythmically, and put the two together. Turning the rope effectively is a skill that must be acquired. Many fitness centers and health clubs have skipping rope specialists. Seek their assistance.

If you are out of shape, start slowly and do not do too much, too soon. In fact, you should first be capable of walking a brisk three miles before you begin a rope skipping program. Be sure to warm up with the Fitness 12 stretching exercises in Chapter 5.

INDOOR FITNESS EQUIPMENT

Last year, Americans spent almost *$1.5 million* on indoor fitness equipment, ranging from $99 for an inexpensive stationary cycle to as much as $10,000 for a motorized treadmill. They have become common in the home, in corporation exercise rooms, and in exercise centers.

Despite the many exercise devices on the market today, developing and maintaining physical fitness does not become easier by using one. William Haskell, Ph.D., an exercise physiologist in preventive medicine at Stanford University Medical School, has observed, "Many people buy a home exercise device hoping it will make exercising easy. When it does not happen that way, the item ends up in the basement or closet."

When deciding what home device to purchase, make sure it will help you exercise most of the large muscles of your body continuously and rhythmically. If rigorous enough, this type of exerceise expends calories, helps increase endurance and muscle tone, and aids cardiorespiratory fitness development.

Using exercise equipment may help some individuals get started, and it provides reasonable alternatives for the walker, runner, cyclist, or swimmer. In the following section we discuss some of the better exercise devices and provide suggestions on how to use such equipment effectively whether at home or at your fitness center.

The Stationary Bicycle

The stationary exercise bike has gained increasing popularity as a convenient means for daily exercise. It is an excellent alternative for people unable to run because of orthopedic problems. It is used in many fitness centers and corporate programs as the main training device. It also serves as an excellent back-up to walking and running workouts. You can listen to the stereo, watch television, or even read a book to help pass the time as you pedal toward fitness!

You can easily develop an effective program using a stationary bike if you understand the principles behind the run-walk-run method of training. The same standards apply. Basically you ride repeated segments of resistance pedaling with short rest periods of no-resistance pedaling or walking around the room. Each workout can be gradually intensified by increasing the length and number of the riding sets as you begin to get in shape.

A good stationery exercise bicycle (often refered to as a cycle ergometer) can be easily adjusted to accurately measure the amount of work being performed as you pedal against a known amount of resistance. Many bikes have built-in timers to assist you in timing your workouts. The cheaper bikes on the market do not accurately measure the amount of work being performed. For the serious exerciser, they leave much to be desired. Fortunately, most fitness centers purchase quality equipment.

If your bike isn't calibrated, you can still use it by measuring your heart rate either during your pedaling or immediately after. This helps regulate the intensity of your effort. The key is to work at your target heart rate whether your bike is calibrated or non-calibrated.

In the privacy of your home, you can wear what you want to wear; however, you do need shoes. To prevent saddle sores, wear shorts with thickness in the seat or put a thick towel across the seat. You are going to perspire so put a pad under the cycle to protect your carpet or flooring.

Make certain your seat is properly adjusted before starting your workout. There should be a slight bend at the knee when your toes are on the pedals with the leg fully extended.

To get accustomed to your bike, pedal for a few days without setting the resistance. Try to pedal at a cadence of one pedal revolution per second or 60 revolutions per minute. When you respond well to this brief introduction, set the resistance up a little and check to see if your exercise effort is challenging enough to elevate your heart rate to a reasonable target for your level of fitness.

You may have to allow some rest periods in between some two-to three-minute rides.

If you are using the bike as an alternative to running, try to duplicate the time and intensity of your run-walk or running program. Even if you have been running continuously for 20 to 30 minutes, you might have to allow some brief rest intervals until your leg muscles are stronger.

Keep a record of your progress and monitor your heart rate to be sure you are putting out enough effort. Your goal is to eventually be able to pedal for 30 minutes or more at your target heart rate at least four times a week.

The Rowing Machine

Rowing exercise machines are becoming very popular. Even for the competitive rower, they serve as good off-water training devices. Some rowing machines now come very close to simulating the rowing of a boat and are quite popular in homes, health clubs, and wellness centers. One particular model, a fly wheel assembly with an electronic monitor, provides an excellent workout. You pull on a chain that rotates the fly wheel. Fan blades built into the fly wheel create wind resistance similar to the water drag on a hull. When you increase the rowing cadence, the wind resistance increases—thus more work is expended.

This indoor exercise machine benefits your heart, lungs, and circulatory system along with providing good exercise for the muscles of your legs, back, shoulders, buttocks, arms, and stomach. A padded seat, shaped like those on rowing shells, lays on ball bearing rollers. An electronic performance monitor calculates the power output and helps you get an accurate read out of your workout.

There are many good rowing devices on the market. Some are highly computerized, combining good durable equipment with video graphics and sound effects to simulate actual rowing competition. Your fitness center specialist can assist you in studying the advantages of one model over another. A workout with the rowing machine is very similar to your walk/run or cycling program. Repeated segments of the rowing with short rest periods represent a good way to get started. As you get in shape, you will be able to row continuously for 30 minutes or more.

The Treadmill

The treadmill, besides being used as a means to test fitness, is used at many fitness centers for exercise training. If you have access to a motorized treadmill, you have an excellent device for walking and running. The walking and running charts adapt easily to treadmill training.

The major disadvantage of a motorized treadmill is the initial cost and operating expense. Costs range from $2,000 to more than $11,000. Before buying one, you should use one at a fitness center or health club. An adjustable-incline treadmill is most helpful for walkers to reach their heart rate target zones.

Climbing and Stepping Machines

New innovative equipment has come on the market that provides vigorous exercise with climbing and stepping movements. Some fitness centers include items in their equipment rooms.

On a climber, you actually simulate the motions of rhythmic climbing. The manufacturers claim that you "exercise all the major muscles with the fastest, safest, most efficient calorie burning, muscle conditioning, and total body workout possible."

These machines are quite unique. Not much testing and research data has been compiled yet. However, you can easily adjust the resistance to regulate your workout. These devices appear to have merit especially for those people who are unable to run.

On the stepping machines, the exercise movement is basic stair climbing. Your body weight is the resistance and the mechanical systems control the speed of movement. This machine and the climber are designed to be the ultimate in low-trauma exercise.

As you contemplate exercising on this equipment, keep in mind our basic principle about exercise training—you must elevate your heart rate into your target zone and maintain this rate over a period of time.

SUMMARY

This chapter by no means describes all the exercise alternatives available to you. Whatever device you may choose, it takes effort to be physically fit. No machine can rub, vibrate, or whirlpool you to fitness. You have to put in the effort.

No matter what exercise program you select, remember to adhere to the guidelines of intensity, duration, and frequency. Make sure your workout is rhythmic and sustaining so you can realize a training effect. Starting out by walking or with an aerobics class may be the catalyst to other fitness activities. As you gain confidence in your abilities and see fitness improvements, you may want to try other fitness ventures.

Part III

Other Fitness Concerns

Another essential segment of your total fitness program is strength and muscular endurance training. Plan to augment your cardio-respiratory moderately intense exercise program with strength-training exercises two or three days a week. Strong, well-toned muscles will help you perform all your sporting activities as well as your daily chores.

Another important aspect of total fitness is maintaining your weight. Good nutrition is the key to building and maintaining strong bones and muscles as well as providing strength to perform all your activities. Chapter 12 provides a primer for nutrition and weight management.

A strong healthy body is ready to engage in other sporting activities and events. The final chapter reinforces an underlying theme of *The Fitness Book* - "You get in shape to play sports."

11

Developing Strength and Muscular Endurance

Strength and muscle endurance help you endure the strains and stresses of daily life. Having reasonably toned and strong muscles will undoubtedly make you more effective in your everyday activities.

Lower back pain, common after the age of 30, is the result of weak abdominal and other trunk muscles. Common remedies for back pain, such as heat application, or even medication, don't get at the primary cause—muscle weakness. Lower back pain can be eliminated or helped by exercising the abdominal and trunk muscles. In fact some experts feel the key to total body fitness is maintaining strong abdominals and trunk muscles.

Whether you walk, run, cycle, swim, or play sports regularly, the chance for injury is always present. Many muscle pulls occur partly because of weakness in either the pulled muscle or its opposing muscle. You need proportional strength. Runners tend to have overdeveloped back leg muscles. Their front leg muscles do not get adequate stimulation. This can cause muscle imbalance and possible injury. Therefore, the front leg muscles need some strengthening to assure better balance. In addition, since walkers, runners, and even cyclists do not get enough arm and shoulder exercises, these body segments need specific strength and endurance exercises.

This chapter provides some basics about developing a strength and muscular endurance program. The idea is not to build large, bulky muscles but to strengthen your muscles to help you to be effective as you engage in your favorite sport or recreation. Integrating strength and muscular endurance training with your cardiorespiratory workout provides you a total approach to fitness.

Strength training is a very important part of your total fitness program. We suggest you spend some additional time on strength training exercises two or three days a week. Strength training and cardiorespiratory endurance go hand-in-hand. Many people starting out on a fitness program do not possess adequate leg strength to walk or run effectively. Therefore exercises to tone and strengthen the large muscle groups need to be incorporated.

It is common today for your personal physician to recommend exercise. In fact, most feel compelled to say something due to the increased general awareness about the benefits of regular exercise. However, through no fault of their own, few physicians understand what proper exercise is. Many have never had any training in this area. Also, many physicians are not active.

Thus, it is safe to suggest walking. It appears harmless, quiet convenient, and requires no instructor. The walking workout as presented in Chapter 6 is productive. But walkers and runners do little in the way of strengthening the major muscle groups. Quite often your heart and lungs are ahead of the muscular and skeletal systems that stimulate them. It is important to give attention to muscular strength and endurance exercises to provide a total program of physical fitness.

This phase of your fitness workout involves activities that tone and strengthen your muscles. Weight training of various types (machines or free weights) or calisthenics like push-ups and abdominal curls provide added muscular strength and endurance needed for you to progress properly in your cardiorespiratory workouts.

Strength is the capacity of a muscle to exert force against a resistance. Endurance is the capacity of a muscle to exert force repeatedly over a period of time or to apply strength and sustain it. It is important to be able to apply force (strength), apply force with speed (power), and be able to sustain this force over a period of time (endurance).

There are two basic types of muscular contractions. *Isotonic* (dynamic) contractions shorten the muscles with a resulting motion: for example, bending your arms as you lift a barbell. *Isometric* (static) contractions are those in which the muscles apply force, but their overall length does not change. Furthermore, movement does not occur. Although there has been some disagreement over the best way to improve strength and endurance, most authorities agree resistance exercises involving movement—isotonic—tend to produce the best results.

WEIGHT TRAINING

One form of isotonic training is accomplished through machines where the resistance follows a fixed path on a cable or chain. This training is referred to as *variable resistance-type* training. Such equipment requires the lifter to exert a maximum effort through a range of movement. Theoretically, this type of equipment provides a greater resistance at the joint angles where you are stronger and a lesser resistance at your weaker positions. The ease of adjusting the weight resistance makes this type of equipment popular and safe.

Such systems as Nautilus, Universal, Eagle, Polaris, and David are examples of variable resistance machines that provide acceptable means for building muscular strength and endurance. The cost of reputable equipment, however, makes it too expensive for most people to buy for personal use. As a result, fitness centers that provide weight training machines have become quite popular. Before you join one, check out the qualifications of the instructors. Most corporate programs employ qualified personnel.

Many fitness trainers still advocate free weights—the use of a bar with weights on the end. The use of free weights is excellent for muscle development, but they require experience. Free weights can also be dangerous. Spotters are required when lifting heavy weights. Get proper instruction so you can learn and develop good technqiue. Small hand weights can also be used safely for muscle toning.

The Overload Principle

A muscle must be overloaded to be strengthened. The development of strength results from an increase in the thickness of the muscle fibers within a muscle—not from an increase in their number! This increase in fiber size is known as hypertrophy.

Generally speaking, the degree of strength improvement in a muscle is directly related to the degree of overload. Once a muscle has adapted to a higher demand, you must give it additional load increases to produce further gains. In weight-resistance exercise (training with barbells and free weights or strength training machines), a muscle is made to contract against a resistance that requires a maximal or near-maximal contraction.

As a rule, lifting against a heavy load (more weight and few repetitions) tends to build maximum strength and muscle size. Lifting less weight with more repetitions tends to build muscular endurance along with good muscular definition and tone. For the average adult, the latter approach for developing strength and endurance is strongly encouraged.

THE EFFECTS OF MUSCULAR DEVELOPMENT IN WOMEN

Both men and women receive beneficial effects from weight-resistance exercise programs. Women normally have less muscle tissue than men. However, among women there is as much variance in muscle mass development as there is among men. Thus, some women are stronger than some men.

The inherent capacity for muscle development is genetically determined by sex hormone levels. The male hormone, testosterone, causes the muscle bulkiness in men. Even though this hormone is present in women, the amount is too low to have a substantial effect on muscle size. In studies that compare the increase in strength of men and women after a period of weight training, women make substantial gains in strength, as do men. However, the muscle size in men increases to almost twice as much as the women's. These findings support the theory that women can increase their strength significantly without a corresponding increase in muscle bulk.

UTILIZING THE FITNESS 12

In Chapter 5, we laid out some exercise primarily aimed at stretching and toning your muscles. If you are unable to use strength training equipment, some of these exercises can be used for muscular development. Increasing the number of repetitions (application of the overload principle) for each exercise can help you improve your strength and muscular endurance. You might also want to consider using small hand and ankle weights for many of the exercises. The arm circles, trunk twister, side stretcher, leg-overs, and the side leg raises are examples of exercises adaptable to small hand or ankle weights.

In addition to the Fitness 12, the sit-up and its variations will strengthen your abdominal muscles, while push-ups will strengthen the muscles in the upper body region.

ABDOMINAL STRENGTHENING EXERCISES

If there is a "must" in every muscular strength and endurance program, it is an exercise to strengthen the abdominals which are difficult to use in many everyday activities. However, these muscles help support the back and various parts of the upper body. They also play a prominent role in maintaining posture and holding in stomachs.

Many experts now believe these muscles are the key foundation for all activity and must be kept in good shape at all times. Biomechanics research has shown that in most activities, force must pass through the center of the body. An athlete or fitness participant who has a weak midsection will be unable to apply the required forces necessary for good performance.

For years, the bent knee sit-up was used extensively. Now researchers suggest variations of the sit-up that are more effective for working and strengthening the abdominals. The following exercises represent ways to strengthen your abdominals and trunk muscles. In all sit-up type exercises it is important that you lift your shoulders before you lift your lower back off the floor.

The Half Sit-Up

Lie on your back with your knees bent at approximately 90 degrees and feet firmly flat on the floor (Figure 11-1). With your arms extended and pointing straight ahead with palms down, raise your shoulders off the floor as you slide your hands up your thighs. Your wrists should go beyond the knees. Lower slowly and relax. Do this six times (Figure 11-1). Rest for one minute. Then repeat two more times after a short rest for a total of three sets.

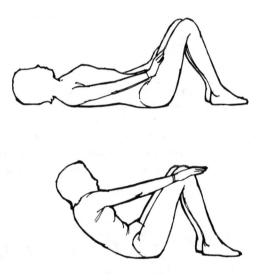

Figure 11-1. The half sit-up.

The Abdominal Cross-over

Lie on your back with left knee bent and left foot flat. Cross the right leg and place the right ankle on the bent knee (Figure 11-2). Put your hands behind your head, elbows out. Avoid pulling on the neck. Curl up and twist your trunk so your left elbow touches your right knee. Lower slowly. Do this six times. Switch and repeat—right elbow to left knee, six times. Do three sets.

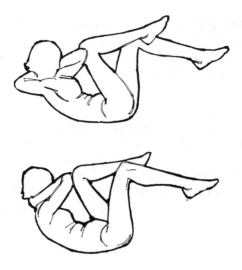

Figure 11-2. Abdominal cross-over.

The Abdominal Curl

Lie on your back with knees bent and feet flat on the floor. Put your hands behind your head, elbows pointing ahead. Avoid pulling on the neck. Raise the bent knees toward the chest so thighs are perpendicular to the floor (Figure 11-3). As you curl up, bring the right elbow toward the left knee. Then bring the left knee back toward the right elbow. Then left elbow to right knee. Repeat this six times to each knee. Do three sets.

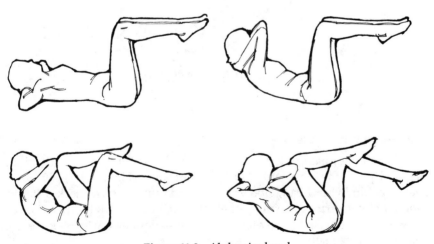

Figure 11-3. Abdominal curl.

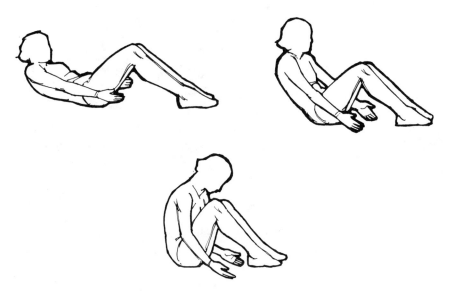

Figure 11-4. Sit-up.

The Full Sit-Up

Lie on your back with knees, feet flat, and arms at your sides. Having someone hold your feet or placing them under a firm support is no longer recommended. Studies show that supporting the feet, even though the knees are bent, tends to involve the large hip flexor muscles more than the abdominals.

A full sit-up entails contracting your abdominals as you curl your back and raise your trunk until your lower back is at least perpendicular to the floor (Figure 11-4). Then lower yourself back to the floor. You may have a problem at first doing a sit-up without support for your feet. It is acceptable to grasp the undersides of your thighs to help pull you up.

As you get stronger, try not to pull on your thighs. By having your hands near your thighs, you will find it easier to balance and curl your trunk to the vertical position.

Do six, rest, repeat two more times.

UPPER BODY STRENGTHENERS

Push-ups represent an old standard for developing the strength in your upper body region. If you cannot even do one, take heart. Many people who have not been exercising lack the strength to do one push-up. The following procedure will help you get started.

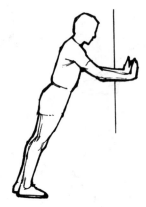

Figure 11-5. Push-away.

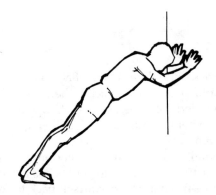

Figure 11-6. Push-away (with hands lower).

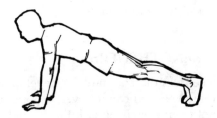

Figure 11-7. Push-up.

Push-Away

Stand with your feet together facing a wall about an arm's length away. Put your hands against the wall at shoulder height. Lean forward until your chest comes near the wall and push back to the starting position (Figure 11-5). Try to repeat the exercise 12 times or until the effort becomes too tough. If you can do 12 repetitions, try another set of 12 after a brief rest. The next day when you work out, try to do 12 push-aways again. As this exercise becomes easier, increase the number of push-aways until you can do two complete sets of 12. Once you can do two sets, then shift your position by moving further from the wall so your hands are lower on the wall, and you are in a more horizontal position (Figure 11-6).

Push-Up

Keep striving to complete two sets of 12 push-aways each day while your hands move lower on the wall. If you find these too easy, then try a stairway or a counter in the kitchen or bathroom. When you find a position where completing 12 push-aways is somewhat tough, then you have found your starting point. Eventually you can put your hands on the floor with your toes in a full push-up position (Figure 11-7.)

As the push-away becomes easier, you increase the resistance to your upper arm and shoulder muscles by putting your body in a position that allows for a greater weight to be moved. You are increasing your strength so you can handle your body weight at least 12 times in a full push-up position. This is a reasonable goal for attaining a minimal amount of upper body strength for men and women. Strive to do 20.

SUMMARY

Keep in mind that a strength training program will firm up muscles, increase muscle tone, and improve body contour and appearance. But, that's all!! Today's research shows strength training does not stress the heart and lungs adequately to improve your cardiorespiratory system. Throughout this book we have emphasized the importance of engaging big muscles in vigorous and rhythmic movements over an extended time period. Running, swimming, brisk walking, rowing, and cycling expend large amounts of energy (calories). Muscles need large amounts of oxygen to produce ample quantities of energy to perform rhythmic endurance-type activities; therefore, a strong cardiorespiratory system is needed to deliver oxygen to the muscle cells. Weight training or similar resistance-type training simply doesn't stimulate the energy systems (oxygen uptake) and the heart sufficiently to bring about significant physiological change.

Nevertheless, a strength and endurance program is important if you want a total fitness workout. However, do not neglect or exclude a cardiorespiratory fitness program in favor of a strength-training program. Having strength and muscular endurance are important—but not at the expense of neglecting your cardiorespiratory training!

12

Weight Management

Eating, although a necessity, is often viewed as a recreation. In a recent Harris survey, 84 percent of those surveyed listed eating as their top leisure-time activity. We snack in front of the TV, at the movies, and at sporting events. We dine at our favorite restaurants, or we invite friends over for dinner. Preparing a tasty meal is a way of showing our affection. Our social routines include holiday feasts, cocktail parties, and backyard barbeques. Business transactions are conducted over food and drink. It is not surprising that 50 percent of all adult Americans are overweight.

Being physically fit also involves maintaining proper body weight. Unfortunately, keeping off excess body fat is a continual struggle for most adults. To most people, the first sign of unfitness is a gain in body weight and increased girth measurements. As a result everyone is looking for a magical, quick way to lose excess weight. Fad diets come and go. However, the importance of exercise and its role in managing your weight is well-established.

A 1986 Harvard School of Public Health study confirms the fatter you are, the sooner you are likely to die. Researchers found individuals living the longest were those who weighed at least 10 percent less than the average for their heights according to the Metropolitan Life Insurance Company's height and weight tables.

Obesity has far-reaching complications. It's closely related to cardiovascular, respiratory, kidney, and gall bladder diseases, as well as diabetes, disorders of bones and joints, and, in some cases, emotional imbalance. Obese people are more prone to fatigue, indigestion, and constipation; they suffer numerous aches and pains. Besides having to cope with the psychological effects of being fat, they face premature death.

Most overweight people don't want to be, so the fight against fat rages on. There are hundreds of weight-reduction plans available. "Fat farms", liposuction, and reducing salons advocate immediate weight loss. Books like *Fit for Life*, *The Rice Diet Report*, and *The Rotation Diet*, continue to be at the top of the bestseller charts. While fad diets may result in temporary weight loss, the weight will eventually return if the dieter learns nothing about changing eating and exercise habits. In fact, according to the American Medical Association, only 5 percent of dieters are successful at loosing excess fat and keeping it off.

In order to treat obesity effectively, we must deal with its causes. We have a proclivity for food, which for most Americans, is plentiful. You need to take in only about 14 more calories than you burn each day to put on a pound and a half in a year. Twenty years later . . . well, you get the picture!

If you are overweight, most likely you've tried your share of diets and exercise programs and have little to show for your efforts—except lost money. Weight management requires time, patience, and effort. No one can do it for you; you can't buy slimness.

How can you lose weight for good? "Lose it slowly," advocates Elliot J. Howard, M.D., a New York cardiologist and author of *Health Risks*. Most people can shed a pound a week by cutting 200 calories a day from their diets (less than two tablespoons of butter) and burning an extra 300 calories daily (a one-hour walk, a 30-minute jog).

YOUR IDEAL WEIGHT

It's not how much you weigh, but rather how much fat you have on your body that determines a proper weight for you. Many people quickly turn to the Metropolitan Life Insurance Company's standard height-weight tables for guidelines. These tables are derived from measurements of a great variety of individuals. Although they enable us to compare ourselves with the average man and woman, they are often inadequate guidelines to ideal weight. Many athletes, low in body fat but very muscular, could be overweight according to these charts. Also, some of these charts allow small increments in body weight with increasing age; this practice lacks justification. Unmistakably, it is the proportion of fat tissue in your body, rather than your scale weight, that determines your proper weight.

A body fat value between 12 to 15 percent of the total body weight is considered trim for adult men; 18 to 22 percent body fat for women. More than 25 percent fat for men and over 30 percent for women indicate obesity.

Most fitness centers, wellness programs, and corporate programs can estimate your body fat with skinfold or other accepted body composition methods. If you are able to pinch up about an inch of fat between your fingers in the flabby areas of your body (Figure 12-1), you have too much body fat.

Genetic Influences

The energy needs of your body depend on your body size, age, and the type and amount of your daily physical activity. We all need the same nutrients, but in different amounts. Young people need greater quantities of food for body growth, upkeep, and energy. Large people need more food than small people. Construction workers need more food than office workers. No matter what your energy needs are, if you take in more calories than you use, you gain weight.

Many people try to claim an abnormal metabolic rate for their obesity, but medical research doesn't support this. Gland malfunction is generally not the reason for obesity.

Researchers have shown that obesity can be caused by genetic factors. However, it is often a result of social or environmental influences.

Recent research indicates the human fat cells increase in number very rapidly in early life; once formed, they become fixed for life. When infants are overfed, they tend to produce more fat cells. This makes weight control more difficult in later life. A fat baby is not necessarily a healthy baby. Preventive steps should be taken at an early age to curb this potential for unnecessarily multiplying an infant's fat cells.

Overfeeding in infancy is often followed by forced feeding in early childhood. Demanding that children clean their plates and using sweets to reward them cultivate bad habits. Sound nutritional habits begin at home.

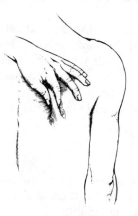

Figure 12-1. Pinch an inch.

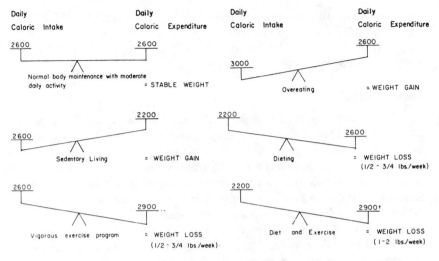

Figure 12-2. Fulcrums.

THE BASIC PRINCIPLE OF WEIGHT CONTROL

The basic principle of weight control is simple. Your energy intake (food) and your energy output (physical activity) must be kept in balance (Figure 12-2). When you eat more than you need for daily energy, the excess energy is stored as body fat. When you eat less, the stored fat is burned for energy. Grasping this principle isn't hard—putting it into practice is!

You must not only watch what you eat, but what you do. In the long run, a strict diet will not be effective unless you become active. Regular exercise with sound eating habits offer the most sensible approach to controlling weight.

The word "diet" is out. Going on and off diets is not the way to manage your body weight. Instead, weight management must be a lifetime activity. Most people with weight problems don't eat too much; they exercise too little. Exercise raises your basic metabolic rate, which helps to burn that stored up fat. The secret to permanent weight control is a combination of sound nutritional principles and an active lifestyle.

NUTRITION BASICS

Nutrition is the study of the food we eat and how our body uses it. Understanding the basics of nutrition will help you in your lifetime commitment to weight management.

Food provides a wide variety of necessary substances, or nutrients. These substances are essential for building and repairing the body as well as for energy. Three basic classes of nutrients are present in the food we eat: proteins, carbohydrates, and fats. Minerals, vitamins, and water are also essential for life but do not provide energy.

Protein

Protein is the basic structural substance of each cell in the body. When we eat, proteins in food are broken down into amino acids. These amino acids travel through the bloodstream and are combined in various parts of the body to form bones, skin, muscle and many organ tissues. Proteins form the structural basis for enzymes and hormones that control and regulate the chemical reactions in the body. Specialized proteins present in the blood serve as clotting agents and oxygen-carrying molecules.

The major sources of protein are foods of animal origin: meat, fish, poultry, eggs and milk. Nutritionists suggest peas, beans, and nuts as good substitutes for animal protein. Approximately 15 percent of our daily caloric intakes should come from protein (Figure 12-3).

Carbohydrates

Carbohydrates—sugar and starches—provide the energy bodies need to form new chemical compounds and to transmit nerve impulses. They also are the primary energy source for muscular activity. (In contrast, proteins are not used significantly for energy during physical activity.) Recommended sources of starches include potatoes, beans, peas, grains (wheat, oats, corn, and rice), flour, pasta, grits, bread, and break-

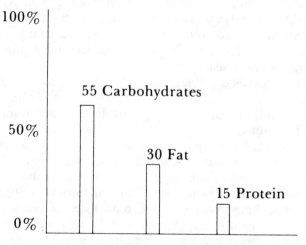

Figure 12-3. Daily calorie consumption.

fast cereal. Sources of sugar are candy, jams, jellies, table sugar, honey, molasses, and concentrated syrups. Fruits, vegetables, and fruit juices also contain fructose. (Sugar, as used in this chapter, refers to sucrose or refined sugar, whereas blood sugar—the end product of carbohydrate breakdown—refers to glucose.)

All carbohydrates serve the same basic purpose: to provide glucose for the body. However, foods containing milk sugar, fruit sugar, and starches are also rich in other essential nutrients.

Sugar must be consumed in moderation and not to the exclusion of other important foods in your diet. Unfortunately the problem with sugar-based foods is they taste so good. The average American consumes well over 100 pounds of refined sugar per year. Much of this sugar is hidden in the processed food we eat regularly. We call them "empty calorie" foods because they provide nothing but energy. Furthermore, overeating sugars may rob your body of the necessary vitamins and minerals. Nutritionist Jean Mayer sums it best: "About the only good thing I can say for sugar is that it tastes good!" Select foods that provide a good nutrient return for the caloric investment.

Approximately 55 percent of your daily caloric intake should come from carbohydrates and 40 percent of that should be carbohydrates other than refined sugar. This means eating more vegetables, fruits, and starches. Whenever you take in more carbohydrates than your body needs, the excess is converted to fat and stored. Hence, a person who eats too many carbohydrate calories is sure to increase the body's fat content.

Fats

The main component of fats—fatty acids—are a concentrated source of energy and provide more than twice as much energy (calories) as comparable amounts of either carbohydrates or protein. Fat is a necessary nutrient. It is an important part of the cell structure; it acts as an insulator and protector of the body's vital parts; and it provides additional energy for muscular activity.

Common sources of fats are fatty meats (bacon, hamburger), butter, margarine, shortening, cooking and salad oils, cream, most cheeses, mayonnaise, nuts, milk, eggs, and chocolate. In addition, anything cooked in fat contains fat.

There are two basic types of fats: saturated and unsaturated. Saturated fats are found in animal products such as meat, milk, cheese, and butter, but are also contained in palm oil, coconut oil and cocoa butter. This type of fat does not melt at room temperature. In contrast, unsaturated fats come from vegetables and tend to be liquid at room temperature. Unsaturated fats are found in peanut and olive oil. Polyunsaturated fats (more liquid) are found in corn, soybean, cottonseed, and particularly, safflower oils.

Research demonstrates that saturated fats raise the cholesterol levels in the bloodstream. Because of this, many nutritionists and physicians are encouraging people to reduce the saturated fats in their diet. Less than 30 percent of your daily caloric intake should come from fats, and saturated fat should be less than 10 percent of total calories. If you reduce your intake of solid fats and use unsaturated or polyunsaturated fats as an alternative to animal fat, you can lower your levels of serum cholesterol.

Cholesterol, a fat-like substance, is found only in animal products, especially egg yolks, liver, brain, shrimp, lobster, and other crustacean foods. Cholesterol is necessary; in fact your body produces some of what it needs. It is required for many of the body's complex functions and is used in making sex hormones. However, when cholesterol levels are too high, deposits can form in the arteries and impair circulation.

Minerals

Calcium, iodine, iron, phosphorous, magnesium, sodium, and potassium are among the minerals that give strength and ridigity to certain body tissues and assist with numerous vital functions.

Calcium is the body's most abundant mineral. It combines with phosphorous to form the teeth and bones. Calcium is also crucial for the normal functioning of muscles. Phosphorus is an essential component for supplying energy to the body. Iodine is an important component of thyroxine, a hormone governing the rate of energy metabolism in the body. Iron is a key component of the hemoglobin in the blood.

Sodium and potassium play key roles in regulating the body's fluid balance. These elements, called electrolytes, are mainly present in the fluids inside and surrounding the cells; they are essential for the proper transmission of nerve impulses. Sodium is present in all living matter, such as meats, poultry, fish, and vegetables. It is added in food processing as a preservative, stabilizer, and taste enhancer. We use sodium chloride—table salt—to flavor our foods. Because sodium can contribute to high blood pressure, physicians strongly recommend limiting its intake. Avoid adding salt to foods and limit your intake of foods containing sodium additives. As a general rule, balanced meals supply all the minerals you need.

Vitamins

Vitamins are organic substances needed for the proper functioning of muscles and nerves. They also play a dynamic role in releasing energy from foods and in promoting normal growth of body tissues. The body's cells cannot form these substances; therefore, vitamins must be provided by the foods you eat.

Some vitamins tend to be retained within the body, stored in fat. Others are transported in the fluids of the tissues and cells and are not stored. The latter vitamins must be consumed in the daily diet; any excessive intake is usually excreted in the urine. Ingesting more vitamins than you need is of limited or no benefit to your body. In fact, excessive intake of vitamins can be harmful. Medical research has documented the toxicity of large doses of vitamins. Healthy people who eat well-balanced meals and a wide variety of foods do not need vitamin supplements.

Water

The body's need for water exceeds its need for food. About three-fourths of your body is water. Water is second only to oxygen in importance. Water transports nutrients and hormones throughout the body and is also essential for removing wastes from the body. Water plays a vital role in regulating body temperature. You get the water you need by drinking it and from the foods you eat.

NATIONAL DIETARY GOALS

The growing recognition of the importance of nutrition in weight management and in the prevention of coronary heart disease has led to the establishment of dietary guidelines for Americans. The 1986 American Heart Association* (AHA) dietary guidelines for healthy American adults are as follows:

1. Saturated fat intake should be less than 10 percent of calories.
2. Total fat intake should be less than 30 percent of calories.
3. Cholesterol intake should be less than 100 milligrams per 1,000 calories, not to exceed 300 milligrams per day.
4. Protein intake should be approximately 15 percent of calories.
5. Carbohydrate intake should constitute 50 to 55 percent of the total caloric intake with emphasis on increasing complex carbohydrates.
6. Sodium intake should be reduced to approximately 1 gram per 1,000 calories, not to exceed 3 grams per day.
7. If alcoholic beverages are consumed, the caloric intake should be limited to 15 percent of total calories.

These guidelines are translatable into a nutritionally, well-balanced diet. If you select a wide variety of foods and prepare them tastefully,

*Available free of charge from the American Heart Association, National Center, 7320 Greenville Avenue, Dallas, Tx. 75231.

you are taking the first step toward adherence to a low-fat, low-cholesterol weight management program.

Caloric Values of Food

Numerous books on diet and nutrition contain long lists of the caloric content of various foods. Since there are often discrepancies in the values of food in diet books, use the *Nutritive Value of American Foods in Common Units* available from the U.S. Department of Agriculture, Washington D.C.

THE ROLE OF EXERCISE IN WEIGHT CONTROL

Physical activity is the great variable in energy expenditure and can play a very important role in helping you maintain your weight. When weight is lost from dieting alone, a significant amount of that loss comes from body water and lean body tissue from the muscles, bones and organs. Many people on low-carbohydrate diets experience quick weight reductions due to loss of body fluid. They are encouraged, yet deceived, by the results. Unfortunately, when the crash diet ends and normal eating resumes, the weight regained will be mostly fat! It takes time to rebuild lean body tissues. When the weight is regained, the dieting often begins again, repeating the process. Constantly going on and off diets can seriously jeopardize one's health.

When beginning exercise programs, many individuals see a gain in lean body weight. This is associated with the build-up of muscle tissue. Even though there is a loss of body fat, total body weight changes little, since the build-up of lean tissue offsets the loss of body fat. This can be discouraging but it should not be. The right kind of weight loss is occurring. After your body adjusts to the new exercise regimen, the build-up of muscle tissue levels off, but the burning off of stored fat continues. This loss will be reflected on the bathroom scale.

Determining Energy Expenditure

When exercise is used for weight reduction, the energy cost of physical activities should be considered in designing a weight-control program. You must determine your energy expenditure in order to balance it with your intake.

The body's expenditure of energy is measured in calories. This energy expenditure is called the caloric cost of an activity. We can calculate the caloric costs by measuring the amount of heat given off by the body. Such measurement is extremely difficult during exercise. However, since heat loss from energy expenditure is related to the amount of oxygen consumed by the body, the rates of oxygen consumption can be used to measure energy expenditure.

Oxygen Caloric Equivalency

One liter (approximately one quart) of oxygen consumed by the body during exercise is equivalent to approximately five calories of expended energy. In other words, one calorie is equivalent to 200 milliliters (0.2 liters) of oxygen consumed. For example, when walking at 3.5 mph, a person of average size (150 pounds) uses about five calories a minute, or 150 Calories in 30 minutes. Since a 12-ounce can of beer contains about 150 calories, it would take 30 minutes of walking to burn off those calories. Clearly, knowing the number of calories in food and the calories you spend in various physical activities can help you embark on a sound weight management program.

Energy Costs of Activities

In recent years much research has been devoted to establishing the energy costs of various sports and exercise activities. When estimating energy expenditure for any individual, we must consider the time spent in the activity, the rate of work, and body size. The more time you spend at an activity, the more energy you use. Larger people tend to require more energy than smaller people for the same task. Table 12-1 describes energy cost during running and walking in calories per minute and in calories per minute per kilogram of body weight. It will enable you to estimate your own caloric costs for selected activities.

Activities requiring five to nine calories per minute (1.0 to 1.8 liters of oxygen) are classified as moderate. Activities requiring above nine calories per minute are classified as vigorous. Table 12-1 presents calorie-per-minute values for running for 120-, 150-, 180-, and 200-pound persons.

Each running speed is expressed in terms of METS, another measure of caloric intensity. A MET refers to the rate of energy expended; one MET is equivalent to the energy needed at rest, or approximately 1.25 calories per minute. Classifying an activity at 7 METS, for instance, means it requires seven times more energy than a state of rest. Seven METS would be at the high end of moderate exercise; it is equivalent to 8.8 calories per minute, or a little more than 1.75 liters of oxygen uptake.

Anything over 10 METs is considered vigorous. Marathon runners run for two to three hours at an intensity level of 14 to 16 METS or more.

How can you estimate your energy cost for walking and running? First determine your body weight in kilograms by multiplying your weight in pounds by .45 (1 pound equals .45 kilogram). Then select your preferred walking or running speed. Multiply your kilogram weight by

Table 12-1. Energy Cost of Walking and Running

	CAL/MIN/KG	CAL/MIN				METS
		120-LB PERSON (54 KG)	150-LB PERSON (68 KG)	180-LB PERSON (81 KG)	200-LB PERSON (90 KG)	RANGE
20-min. mile (3 mph)	0.0577	3.1	3.9	4.6	5.2	2.5 to 4
17.5-min. mile (3.4 mph)	0.0692	3.7	4.7	5.6	6.2	3 to 5
15-min. mile (4 mph)	0.0872	4.7	5.9	7.1	7.8	4 to 6
10-min. mile (6 mph)	0.1471	7.9	10.0	11.9	13.2	6 to 11
8-min. mile (7.5 mph)	0.1856	10.0	12.6	15.0	16.7	8 to 13
7-min. mile (8 mph)	0.2118	11.4	14.4	17.2	19.1	9 to 15
6-min. mile (10 mph)	0.2350	12.7	16.0	19.0	21.2	10 to 17

the value under the column headed cal/min/kg in the energy table. This will be the caloric cost per minute for you.

$$\underline{\hspace{3cm}} \quad \times \quad .45 \quad = \quad \underline{\hspace{3cm}}$$

| Your body weight in pounds | | Your body weight in kilograms |

$$\underline{\hspace{3cm}} \quad \times \quad \underline{\hspace{3cm}} \quad = \quad \underline{\hspace{3cm}}$$

| walk/run speed cal/min/kg (from chart) | Your weight in kilograms | Your caloric cost/ minute |

Compare two men, both weighing 68 kilograms. One can run four miles in 28 minutes (a seven-minute-mile pace) at a heart rate of 150 (an adequate training stimulus). The other can run 2.8 miles during the same period (28 minutes at a 10-minute-mile pace) and at the same heart rate. The first runner utilizes 403 calories for his workout; the second man utilizes only 280 calories during his workout. We can readily see the man in better physical condition burns more calories during a 28-minute workout than the slower runner. This means more calories expended—a bonus for weight control.

Now let's assume the slower runner runs a total distance of four miles; he would then use another 120 calories, which would give him a similar caloric expenditure, 400 calories. But his total workout time is 40 minutes rather than 28. The runner who can run the four miles in 28 minutes has a greater functional fitness capacity than the slow runner. Nevertheless, for burning calories to control or maintain your weight, the most important factor is the distance you move, not the speed at which you move.

Table 12-2 presents caloric (energy) values for selected sports activities. We have arranged the table in ascending order from the less intensive activities to a more intense activity.

Sports like golf and bowling do not represent a suitable means for developing or maintaining physical fitness. They do not put enough stress on the cardiorespiratory system to produce training effects. For weight control, however, these sports can be beneficial. Although the cardiorespiratory stimulation is minimal, extra calories are burned. If we compare the 150-pound person who runs four miles in 28 minutes to a golfer of the same weight, we find the golfer must play for a total of 106 minutes to burn the same 403 calories. To put this another way, the golfer has to play nearly four times as long as the runner has to run for the same energy-cost benefits.

Table 12-2. Energy Cost of Selected Sporting Activities

	CAL/MIN/KG	CAL/MIN*	METS*
Bowling (with three other bowlers)	0.0471	3.2	2.6
Golf (playing in a foursome)	0.0559	3.8	3.0
Walking (17.5-min. mile)	0.0692	4.7	3.8
Cycling (6.4-min. mile)	0.0985	6.7	5.4
Canoeing (15-min. mile)	0.1029	7.0	5.6
Swimming (59 yd/min.)	0.1333	9.1	7.3
Running (10-min. mile)	0.1471	10.0	8.0
Cycling (5-min. mile)	0.1559	10.6	8.5
Handball (singles)	0.1603	10.9	8.7
Rope skipping (80 turns/min.)	0.1655	11.3	9.0
Running (8-min. mile)	0.1856	12.6	10.1
Running (6-min. mile)	0.2350	16.0	12.8

*These are values for a 150-pound person (68 kg).

COMMON MISCONCEPTIONS

Misconceptions about the relationship between exercise and weight control are quite common. Here are a few of them:

Exercise and Appetite

Often we hear the phrase "the more you exercise, the more you will eat." Mayer has concluded that a daily exercise session does not bring about a corresponding increase in appetite and food intake. Appetite is a fairly good guide to the amount of food needed by active people, but it is not a reliable measure for inactive people. Therefore, it does not follow if you are inactive you will eat less than if you are active. He suggests there is a range of inactivity where the food intake no longer correlates with a decrease in activity. In that range, there is an imbalance between food intake and energy output—and fatness results. Mayer calls this the "sedentary range." Above this range of inactivity is the range of normal activity, where appetite and exercise are attuned to each other.

Spot Reducing

Health spas and weight-reducing salons often promote spot reducing programs. Women are frequently encouraged to use localized exercise or mechanical vibrators and other gadgets to reduce the fatty stores in areas where they have greater fat deposition. Research has shown, however, exercise or massaging a particular area of the body will not reduce the excess fat in the region. Calisthenics, yoga, or slimnastics are beneficial to general muscle tone and flexibility. They do not, however, spot reduce.

Several studies have shown vigorous, regular, and continuous exercise involving total body movement does reduce skinfold fat and girth measurements. When fat is reduced, it tends to be reduced all over the body, in proportion to the amount present at any given site. Muscles do not use the fat stored near them. Instead, hormone signals go to the fat storage deposits throughout the body. These cells release fat molecules into the blood stream. The blood takes them to the working muscle to be used as fuel.

Weight Reduction by Sweating

Many people hope that overheating their bodies will cause a quick loss of excess body weight. Exercising in hot, humid weather or while wearing a rubber sweat suit are common methods for prompting profuse sweating. Granted, the scales may read a pound or two lower, but the weight loss has nothing to do with body fat, and it will not be permanent.

Basically, sweating procedures accomplish only one thing—a greater-than-normal loss of water from the body. If excessive, this water loss can cause serious problems. A rubber suit or any unneeded clothing in hot, humid weather does not allow the heat produced during exercise to escape from the body. Sweat evaporation is the major means for dissipating heat at the skin's surface during vigorous exercise. When you wear a rubber suit, the trapped sweat can't evaporate to cool the body.

Eventually the body heat is raised beyond its normal range, imposing an added burden on the body. This leads to a loss of too much body water and, in turn, a decrease in blood volume, a severe rise in body temperature, and possible circulatory collapse. These events, if severe enough, can produce heat stroke and death.

Dehydration (removal of body water) is useless for weight control and can be dangerous. You immediately restore the depleted body water when you eat and drink. Water does not contain calories. Excess body weight (fat) is only lost by burning calories, not by losing water.

A PLAN FOR LOSING WEIGHT

Weight control is a lifetime concern, not a two-week special diet. Don't embark on a diet you're not willing to follow for life! Exercising allows you to burn an extra 300 to 500 calories or more each workout.

That will help you lose excess fat and help you keep it off. Once you reach your desired weight, you can eat more than inactive people without gaining weight—if you remain physically active.

Setting Goals

Before you begin a weight loss program, set up some realistic targets. Determine the number of pounds you need to lose, the number of weeks it will take, and the maximum number of calories you should eat every day. It is helpful to make a chart or a graph indicating your beginning weight and your final desired weight loss. Put the chart on your refrigerator or somewhere in the kitchen or bathroom for handy reference.

First, determine your ideal or desired weight. Regardless of how you determine your ideal weight, subtract this target value from your present weight. The result is the number of pounds to lose.

Weight reduction should be gradual, at a rate of no more than two pounds per week. If you divide the number of pounds you want to lose by one (or two) pounds, this will give you the number of weeks needed to reach your desired weight. No doubt it will be longer than you would like, but if you stick to this realistic plan, you'll never see these pounds again, if you remain physically active.

You will also have to determine the maximum daily caloric intake possible to enable you to lose your targeted number of pounds. Most moderately-active people need about 15 calories per pound per day to maintain their weight. If you are moderately active, multiply your present weight by 15 to determine the number of calories needed for your daily activities. If you are inactive, a more realistic value is 12 calories per pound of body weight. If you are quite active, a value of 18 calories is reasonable for figuring your daily caloric needs.

There are approximately 3,500 calories in each pound of stored fat. To lose one pound a week, you must reduce your caloric intake by 500 calories a day. Therefore, for the 190-pound, moderately active person, this means cutting the number of daily calories from 2,850 to 2,350. Given today's choice of readily available foods, this can be difficult. That is why becoming more active in a regular exercise program can be the key to losing weight permanently.

Making It Easier Through Vigorous Exercise

It requires an energy expenditure of 3,500 calories to lose a pound of fat. Even if you exercised very vigorously for 30 minutes, you would be hard pressed to burn 500 calories. Very few people have this capability, especially when beginning an exercise program. But, if you take a long-range view and exercise at a more reasonable caloric level of 300 calories for four days a week, you could burn an extra 1,200 calories a week. Therefore, if you maintain your food intake at a constant level and exercise four days a week, you would lose about one pound every three weeks, or 17 pounds a year!

Now, if you combine vigorous exercise with a cutback of calories, your ability to shed excess pounds increases. Again, if you exercise four days a week at 300 calories per session and cut your daily food intake by 400 calories (that's two cans of beer and a handful of peanuts), you have a 4,000 calories deficit per week. Theoretically, this approach would result in a weight loss of approximately one pound of fat a week.

Before you decide that this one or two pounds a week is too slow, remember, you did not put this weight on overnight, and you are not going to take it off permanently overnight. If your weight is going to stay off, the process must be slow.

Throughout this book, a strong case has been made for the importance of vigorous exercise both for your cardiorespiratory system and weight management. If you are overweight and have been inactive, use the walking charts in Chapter 6. Once you can walk 45 minutes to an hour, you will be burning close to 300 calories or more. As you become more fit and can increase the intensity of your workouts, the more calories you can burn.

To put it more simply—proper exercise on a regular basis is the best way to achieve lifelong weight management.

Special Diets

For some people it helps to follow a planned diet. Others find it helpful to work with a registered dietitian or other nutrition specialist.

Stay away from severe caloric restrictions and be suspicious of diets eliminating essential nutrients. Many people have joined Weight Watchers International® and have benefited from its weekly motivational sessions and diet plans. While these programs might help you at first, eventually you must learn to manage your personal nutritional habits. Although we do not like the word "diet," a planned program of eating may be necessary to start you on a weight control program. You will find, as in using the exercise charts, you won't need to follow a planned diet every day. Your exercise and eating habits will become an integral part of your everyday living.

Changing Your Lifestyle

There's no magical formula or easy way to lose weight. It's hard work to change eating patterns and include exercise in your life.

The following pointers are recommended:

1. Become more active—begin an exercise program. Believe it or not, there are thousands of formerly fat people walking, swimming, jogging, and skiing today.

2. After you have embarked on an exercise program, begin making dietary changes.

3. Observe your eating habits for a week or two. Write down what you eat, when, where, and how much. Then ask yourself why you ate it. Reading a diary at the end of the week may surprise you. Understanding your eating habits is half the battle.

4. Separate your eating from other behaviors. Don't eat on the run, in front of the TV, or in the bedroom. When you eat—eat. Don't do anything else while you enjoy your food.

5. Put a serving of food on your plate. Then put away leftovers before you sit down. This makes it tougher to get extra helpings.

6. Buy groceries on a full stomach. This prevents impulse buying. Don't buy junk foods you crave.

7. Eat slowly. Slowing down gives your digestive system time to let your brain know food is being received. It takes about 20 minutes for food to get into your blood stream and turn off your hunger pangs.

8. Make weight management a family affair.

The human body was made to be active. It thrives on movement and vigorous activity. The ability to sit all day without getting fat was not bred into our bodies.

A sound, nutritious diet combined with regular vigorous exercise is the best strategy for a lifetime of successful weight control. The goal is not merely to lose fat, but to keep it off. Better still, never put it on.

13

Get In Shape For Sports

Throughout this book we have stressed the importance of regular exercise as the key to total well-being. We are confident that if you follow the exercise guidelines for achieving and maintaining fitness as presented, you can look forward to many years of robust health and good living.

Being fit also opens up more opportunities for you to get involved in sports. Many of us need more reasons than physiological health to keep us motivated to exercise regularly. It is not surprising to find that people who are physically active are driven by the desire to be in shape to participate in various sporting activities. Our experiences reveal people who started out exercising just to get in shape and lose some weight are now training to run, sail, ski, or play racquetball.

It is our firm belief that *sports are played for fun, not for fitness.* It has been traditionally assumed that playing sports is a way of keeping in shape. For many years physical educators, coaches, and even athletes have operated under the mistaken notion that you can "play yourself" into good condition. This thesis sounds reasonable, but we now know that a certain amount of basic conditioning is needed to supplement most athletic and sports programs. Athletes now train with weights, and they run regularly. They are more knowledgeable about training, injury prevention, and nutrition. The same should be true for the average sports participant. *You need to get in shape to play sports, rather than play sports to get in shape.* Whether you are participating in triathalons or the local softball league, being in good physical shape will help to prevent injury and, most importantly enjoy your sport to the fullest.

Running or swimming laps may become somewhat monotonous. But anyone active in a sport finds such training acceptable when its purposes include not only good health and fitness, but also better preparation for actual play. Whatever your preference—tennis, golf, skiing, or basketball—you will enjoy these activities more if you keep your body in firm muscular and cardiorespiratory shape through a program of fitness training.

RATING THE FITNESS POTENTIAL OF LIFETIME SPORTS

Most sports—team or individual—do not provide sufficient endurance-type movement to develop and maintain cardiorespiratory fitness. But, participation in some sports can complement your overall fitness conditioning program. Sports that require speed, quick movements, and strength provide an important dimension to your all-around fitness development. However, maintaining regular muscular strength and endurance workouts along with flexibility routines can assure better preparation for playing sports.

Keep in mind that the benefits from sports participation vary from person to person. Any attempt to rate and compare the sports as to their relative contribution to developing physical fitness can be questioned. To date, there is only limited research to support such judgments. The intensity of a player's activity and the energy required varies according to age, skills, and fitness level, and in team sports, the skill of other players. Therefore the energy cost values for sports are not as exact as we would like. Nevertheless, we have developed Table 13-1, which includes energy cost ratings that are based on our own as well as others' research. For each sport listed, we give a MET range and a range of estimated caloric values. The exact amount of energy (calories) depends on how much you weigh as well as how vigorously you play. Qualifying words (i.e., excellent, good, fair, poor) as to the overall potential of each sport as a fitness developer are provided to help you to make comparisons. What is most important is how demanding these sports are on the body. In other words, what are the specific physiological requirements of each?

For an example, look at racquetball. It is a sport that most people can play with reasonable success after brief instruction and practice. How does it rate as a fitness activity? Racquetball is vigorous; it uses big muscles; it requires high levels of energy and, it is generally played for at least an hour. It is not played continuously but intermittently with brief stops in between serves. Successful play is highly dependent on the functional ability of your heart and aerobic systems. It does require strength, particularly the ability to sustain strength—muscular endurance. Range of motion-flexibility is quite specific as similar muscular movements are repeated constantly. Therefore, as the chart indicates, racquetball rates good on cardiorespiratory endurance, muscular strength and endurance (upper and lower body), and fair to good on flexibility. Keep in mind these ratings are based on the average partici-

162   THE FITNESS BOOK

Table 13-1. Fitness Potential For Popular Sports

SPORT	CARDIO-RESPIRATORY ENDURANCE	MUSCULAR STRENGTH & ENDURANCE		FLEXIBILITY	MET RANGE	CAL/MIN	CALORIC RANGE CAL/HOUR
		UPPER BODY	LOWER BODY				
Back packing[1]	Good to Fair	Fair	Good	Fair	4-8	5-10	300-600
Badminton	Good to Fair	Fair	Fair	Fair	4-8	5-10	300-600
Baseball/Softball	Fair to Poor	Fair	Fair	Fair	3-6	4-7.5	240-450
Basketball	Good	Fair	Good	Fair	8-10	10-12.5	600-750
Bowling	Poor	Fair	Poor	Poor	2-3	2.5-4	150-240
Canoeing	Good to Fair	Good	Poor	Poor	3-8	4-10	240-600
Football (touch)	Fair to Poor	Fair	Fair	Fair	4-8	5-10	300-600
Golf	Poor	Fair	Good	Fair	3-4	4-5	240-300
Handball	Good	Good	Good	Fair	6-12	10-12.5	600-750
Karate	Fair	Good	Good	Excellent	6-8	7.5-10	450-600
Racquetball	Good	Good	Good	Fair	6-10	7.5-12.5	450-750
Scuba diving	Poor	Fair	Fair	Fair	4-6	5-7.5	300-450
Skating (ice)	Good to Fair	Poor	Good-Fair	Fair	4-8	5-10	300-600
Skating (roller)	Good to Fair	Poor	Good-Fair	Fair	4-8	5-10	300-600
Skiing (alpine)	Fair	Good	Good	Good	5-9	6-10	360-600
Skiing (nordic)	Excellent-Good	Good	Excellent	Good	6-12	7.5-15	450-900

Table 13-1. Cont.

SPORT	CARDIO-RESPIRATORY ENDURANCE	MUSCULAR STRENGTH & ENDURANCE		FLEXIBILITY	MET RANGE	CAL/ MIN	CALORIC RANGE CAL/HOUR
		UPPER BODY	LOWER BODY				
Soccer	Good-Excellent	Fair	Good-Excellent	Good	6-12	7.5-15	450-900
Surfing[2]	Good[2]	Good	Good	Good	4-10	5-12.5	300-750
Tennis	Good-Fair	Good-Fair	Good	Fair	4-8	5-10	300-600
Volleyball	Good-Fair	Fair	Good-Fair	Fair	4-8	5-10	300-600
Waterskiing	Poor	Good	Good	Fair	4-6	5-7.5	300-450

[1]Benefits depend on walking terrain and weight of pack.
[2]Paddling the board out beyond the breaking waves can be demanding.

pant rather than the expert player. Generally the energy required to play racquetball properly can range from as low as eight METs to as high as 12 METs. The reason for this wide range is the variance of both the skill and the fitness capabilities of the participant. To put it another way, eight METs, when expressed as maximal fitness, is considered low for active people. One needs a 10- or 11-MET max to be able to perform an activity at an 8 MET level. On the other end of the scale, if you are capable of playing racquetball at a 12-MET level, this requires a high fitness capacity of 15 to 16 METs.

This example further clarifies the point that *you need to get in shape so you can play to the fullest your favorite sport*. The better your condition, the better your chance of getting a good workout when playing sports. If you presently possess a low level of fitness, investing significant amounts of time playing racquetball or any other sport for developing fitness is questionable. First, involve your total body in sustained vigorous exercise so you can develop your heart, lungs, and muscles so you fully enjoy the maximal benefits from sports participation.

Index

Metropolitan Life Insurance Company Tables, 143, 144
METs, 152-155, 162-165
Minerals, 149
Mode: of exercise program, 47
Muscle, 6; build-up of, 151; contractions of, 8, 134; development, 22; endurance, 6, 8, 10, 24, 38, 41-43, 51; injuries, 91; overload, 135, 136; size in women, 135-136; strength, 133-142; stretching, 91, 94; tone, 89, 133, 141; weakness, 133

National Institute of Health, 27
Neuromuscular skill, 6
Nutrition, 146-147

Obesity, 9, 143-144
Optimal physiological health, 10
Orthopedic doctor, 81
Oxygen: consumption rates, 151-152; uptake, 25-26

Paffenbarger, Ralph S., 22
Phosphorus, 149
Podiatrist: sports, 81
Potassium, 149
President's Council on Physical Fitness and Sports, 106
Proteins, 147, 150
Pulse rate, 48, 49, 80, 83
Push-away, 141
Push-ups, 8, 42-43, 139-141

Racquetball, 162-163, 165
Respiratory system, 13
Rope skipping, 125, 155
Rowing machine, 127-128
Running, 87, 133, 134; apparel for, 88-89; calories consumed in, 152-155; charts for, 92-102; heart rate during, 90; injuries, 91; locations for, 88; mechanics of, 89-90; tests, 39

Scuba diving, 163
Self-testing: fitness, 38-45
Shin splints, 91, 103
Side and groin stretcher, 64
Side leg raises, 66
Sit and reach test, 44
Sit-ups, 8, 41-42, 136-137, 138
Skating, 163
Skiing, 164, 165
Smith, Everett, 22
Smoking, 11, 30
Soccer, 164
Sodium, 149, 150
Sorenson, Jackie, 123
Stamina, 6
Standing quad stretcher, 73
Stationary cycling, 126-127
Stepping machines, 128
Strength, 6-8, 24, 38; definition of, 134; development of, 51, 133-142; lack of, 8; tests of, 41-43
Stress, 5, 30
Stretching, 57-74, 91, 94, 107, 117, 125
Stride stretcher, 71
Submaximal tests, 38

Sugar, 147-148
Surfing, 164
Sweating, 156
Swimming, 103; apparel for, 104; calories consumed in, 155; charts for, 107-112; intensity of, 105-106; locations for, 104; strokes, 105
Swimnastics, 106
Systolic pressure, 18-20, 37

Target heart rate, 49-50, 52-53, 80, 83
Tendinitis, 91
Tennis, 164
Testosterone, 22, 136
Thigh muscles, 43
Three-segment workout, 50-51
Toning exercises, 57-74
Trachea, 14, 16
Treadmill, 35-36, 128
Triglycerides, 27, 36
Trimness, 6, 9
Trunk flexion test, 43
Trunk twister, 63

United States Centers for Disease Control, 4

Ventricles, 13-14
Vitamins, 149-150
Volleyball, 164

Walking, 77-85, 87, 133, 134; calories consumed in, 152-155; charts, 81-85; tests, 38-39
Warm-up, 50-52, 57-74
Water, 150, 156
Weight: control of, 28, 143-144, 146, 151-154, 155-159; ideal, 9, 144-145, 157
Weight training, 134-135
Weight Watchers International®, 158
Wellness continuum, 3-4
World Health Organization, 30

YMCA, 11, 38
YWCA, 11, 38
Yoga, 156